Hartkop, David T.

Create a Temperature Controlled Vaccine & Insulin Cooler

Kindle Direct Publishing ISBN: 9781070454603

For more information write to:

Idea Propulsion Systems
4070 Willow Springs Rd.
Central Point OR 97502

Table of Contents

Introduction

Keeping cool saves lives

In the developing world, vaccines are the front line of defense against dangerous illnesses such as Ebola, Influenza, Cholera, Tuberculosis and Dengue to name a few. Transporting vaccines and other life-saving materials such as insulin and blood require careful temperature control.

First-world logistics tend to break down when supplies are transported into regions with limited resources. Many rural medical clinics lack the funding or the energy for ordinary refrigeration systems. Insulin, human blood, and many common vaccines must be kept in the temperature range of 2-8 ℃. In the field, this can be difficult to maintain because electric refrigeration requires too much power, and passive ice coolers lack thermostat control.

Arduino to the rescue

This project combines the compact cooling power of dry-ice (solid carbon dioxide) with the precision of digital temperature control. When used by itself, dry ice too cold to transport vaccine, insulin or blood because it can easily lead to freezing. This project's cooler design solves the problem of freezing by placing the dry ice in a separate chamber below the cargo cooler. A brushless PC fan is used to circulate small doses of super-chilled air through the cargo section as needed. This fan is controlled by a robust Arduino microcontroller, running a temperature control loop. Because the Arduino system runs on very little electrical power, this system can be mobile like an ice chest, but temperature-regulated like a plug-in refrigerator.

Who is this project for?

This project is designed to be built by students, engineers, and aid workers in or near areas facing humanitarian challenges. The materials, parts, and supplies are generally available in most of the world's cities in even the poorest countries. By making the plans available for free, we are providing technology with flexibility in terms of cost and scalability. The decentralized manufacture of these arduino-ice coolers may be in important option with the potential to save lives.

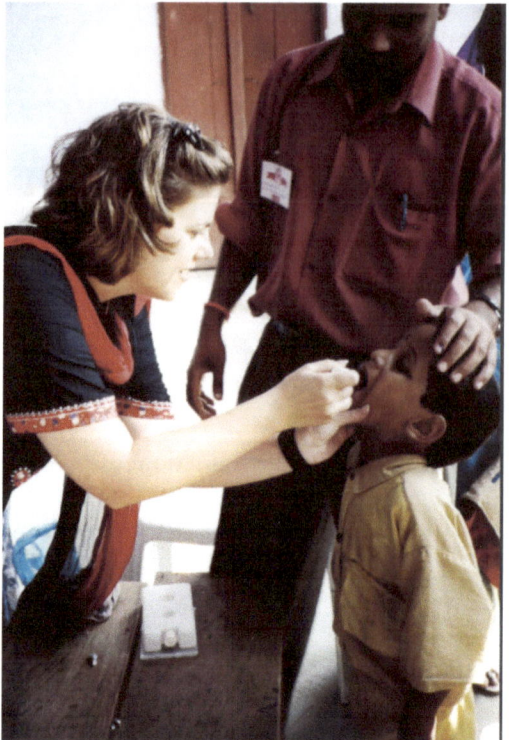

Polio vaccination in India - Photo Credit: Centers For Disease Control and Prevention

Finished cooler specifications:

• Cargo volume: Maximum 6.6 gallons (25L), recommended 5 gallons (19L) with buffer bottles.

• Maximum cargo volume dimensions: =~14 in x 14 in x 8 in (35.6 cm x 35.6 x 20.3 cm)

• Cooling Capacity: Maintains 5°C for 10-7 days in 20-30°C ambient environment respectively.

• Power source: Dry ice and flooded 12 volt marine cell battery.

• Over all dimensions: 24in x 24 in x 32 in tall (61 cm x 61 cm x 66.6 cm tall)

• Over all weight: 33.3 lb (15.1 Kg) empty with no ice / 63 lb (28.6kg) with full ice and cargo.

• Temperature regulation: PID control maintains 5°C +-0.5°C

• Materials: construction grade closed-cell foam and construction adhesives with IR reflective insulation jacketing.

Create a Temperature Controlled Vaccine & Insulin Cooler

Step 1: Setup for the project

Workspace

This project requires some cutting and gluing of styrene foam insulation. This can produce some dust, especially if you opt to use a saw rather than a knife. Be sure to use a dust mask. Also, it is very useful to have a shop-vac on hand to clean up the dust as you go.

Construction adhesive can release irritating fumes when drying. Be sure to complete the gluing and caulking steps in a well ventilated area.

Assembling the arduino add-on components requires the use of a soldering iron. Use lead-free solder when possible, and be sure to work in a well lighted, well ventilated space.

All tools

- Circular saw or scoring knife
- Cordless drill with 1.75 inch hole saw bit
- Soldering iron & solder
- Lighter or heat gun
- 4-foot straight edge
- Sharpie marker
- Ratchet straps
- Tape measure
- Caulking tube dispenser
- Wire cutter/Strippers
- Screwdrivers large and small phillips & regular

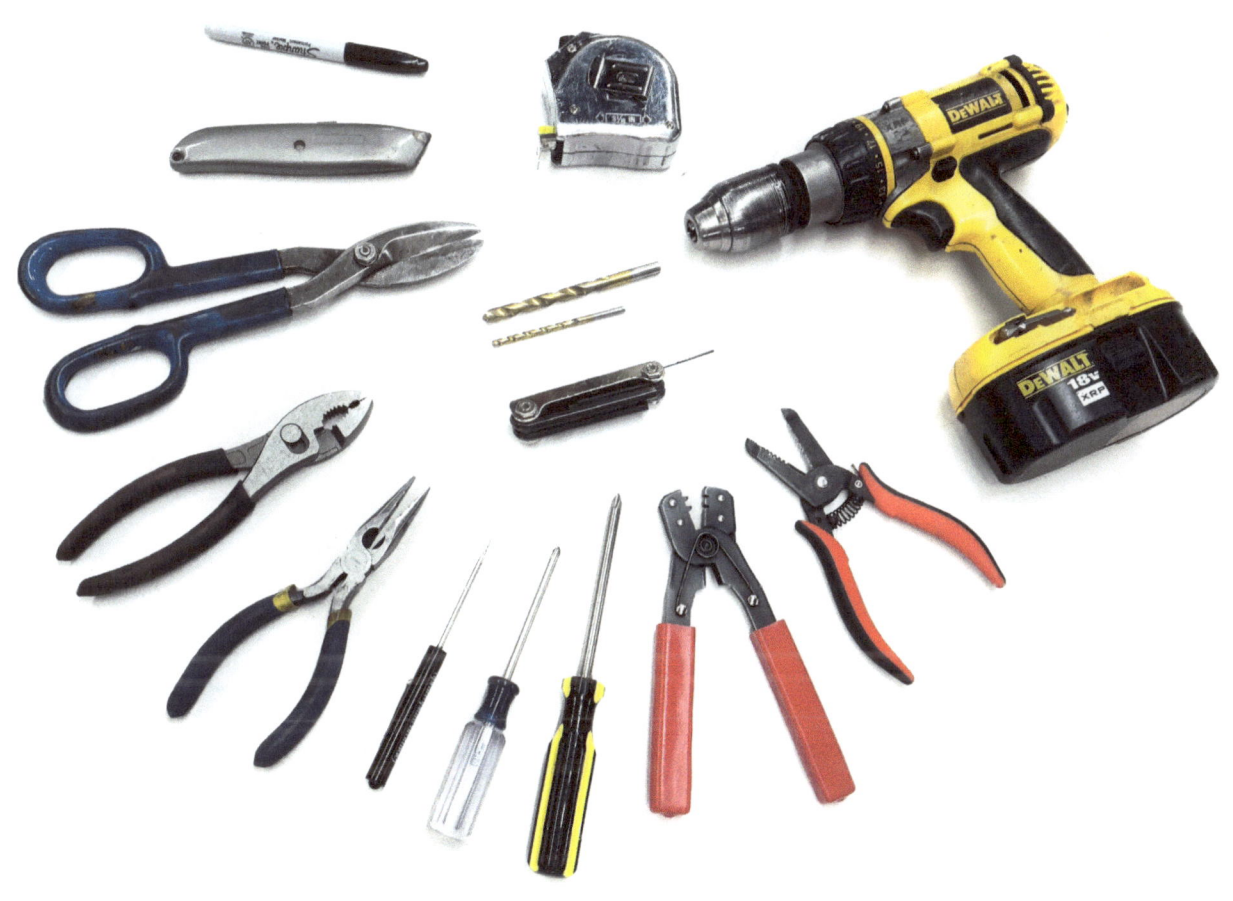

Create a Temperature Controlled Vaccine & Insulin Cooler

All supplies:

Electronics Supplies
• Shrink Tubing 1/8 and 1/4 inch

• Circuit board pin headers (female sockets and male pins)

• ABS plastic electrical box with clear cover, size 7.9"x4.7"x2.94" (200mmx120mmx75mm)

• Rechargable sealed lead acid battery, 12V 20AH. Search for 'NPP HR1280W' or similar.

• Arduino Uno R3 microcontroller board or similar

• Arduino stackable prototype board: Alloet mini breadboard prototype shield V.5 or similar.

• MOSFET driver module IRF520 or similar

• Digital temperature sensor DFRobot DS18B20 in waterproof cable package

• Brushless 12V PC cooling fan: 40mm x 10mm 12V 0.12A

• Micro SD card reader: Adafruit ADA254

• Realtime clock: DIYmore DS3231, based on DS1307 RTC

• Battery for realtime clock: LIR2032 coin cell)

• 4.7 K-ohm resistor

• 26 gauge stranded hook-up wire spools (Red, Black, Yellow)

• Length of 2-conductor speaker wire (3 ft or 1m) 12 gauge stranded (battery hook up wire)

• Automotive blade fuse holder and 3 amp blade fuse (for use with battery)

• USB printer cable (type a male to b male)

• Wire nuts (12 gauge)

Tapes & Adhesives Supplies
• High-adhesion utility tape 2 inch wide x 50 ft roll (Gorilla Tape or similar)

• Silicone caulk, one tube

• Construction adhesive, 2 tubes. (Liquid Nails or similar)

• Aluminum furnace tape, 2 inch wide x 50 ft roll.

• Self adhesive hook-and-loop strips (1 inch wide x 12 inches total needed)

Construction Materials Supplies
• 2 x 4 foot x 8 foot x 2 inch thick (1200 mm x 2400 mm x 150 mm) foam insulation sheets

• 2 ft x 25 ft roll of double reflective air roll furnace insulation, silver bubble.

• 2 x short PVC Pipes, 1 1/2 inch inner diameter x Sch 40. cut to 13 inch lengths.

• Specialty Supplies
Vaccine thermometer:"Thomas Traceable Refrigerator/

• Freezer Plus Thermometer with Vaccine Bottle Probe' and traceable calibration certificate or similar.

• 2 x Flower-stem bottles for liquid-buffering the DS18B20 waterproof temperature probes.

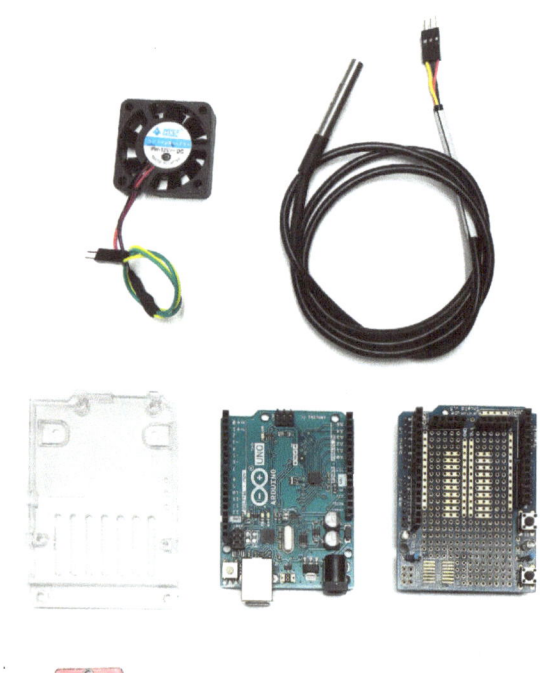

 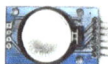

3

Step 2: Cut out the foam parts

Print out the cut-pattern, which shows a number of rectangles to cut from two 4 ft x 8 ft x 2 in (1200 mm x 2400 mm x 150 mm) sheets of rigid closed cell foam insulation.

Foam Sheet #1

22" x 16" 559mm x 406mm	22" x 16" 559mm x 406mm
22" x 16" 559mm x 406mm	22" x 16" 559mm x 406mm
22" x 22" 559mm x 559mm	22" x 22" 559mm x 559mm
18" x 18" 457mm x 457mm	18" x 18" 457mm x 457mm

14" x 14"
356mm x 356mm

14" x 14"
356mm x 356mm

10" x 10"
254mm x 254mm

Foam Sheet #2

| 20" x 26"
508mm x 660mm | 20" x 26"
508mm x 660mm |
| 20" x 26"
508mm x 660mm | 20" x 26"
508mm x 660mm |

12" x 8"
305mm x 203mm

12" x 8"
305mm x 203mm

12" x 8"
305mm x 203mm

12" x 8"
305mm x 203mm

Cut-Pattern for Temp. Controlled Vaccine & Insulin Cooler
Cut from two X 4 ft x 8 ft x 2 inch thick (1200mm x 2400 mm x 150mm) sheets of closed cell rigid construction foam insulation.

4

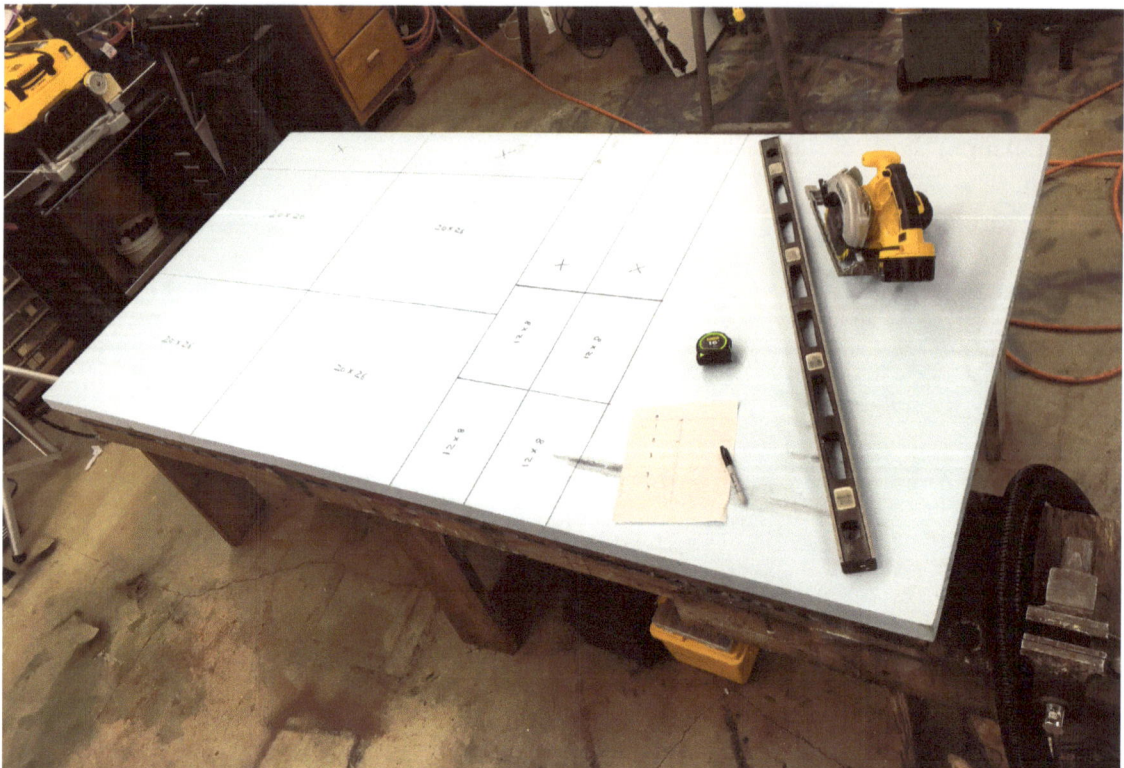

Use a straight edge and marker to carefully draw the lines for cutting the foam sheets. The foam may be cut by scoring it with a utility knife, but it is easiest to use a circular saw to do the job. Cutting foam with a saw, however, produces dust that should not be inhaled.

Precautions:
• Wear a dust mask.

• Use a vacuum hose attached to the saw for dust collection.

• Do the cutting outside if possible.

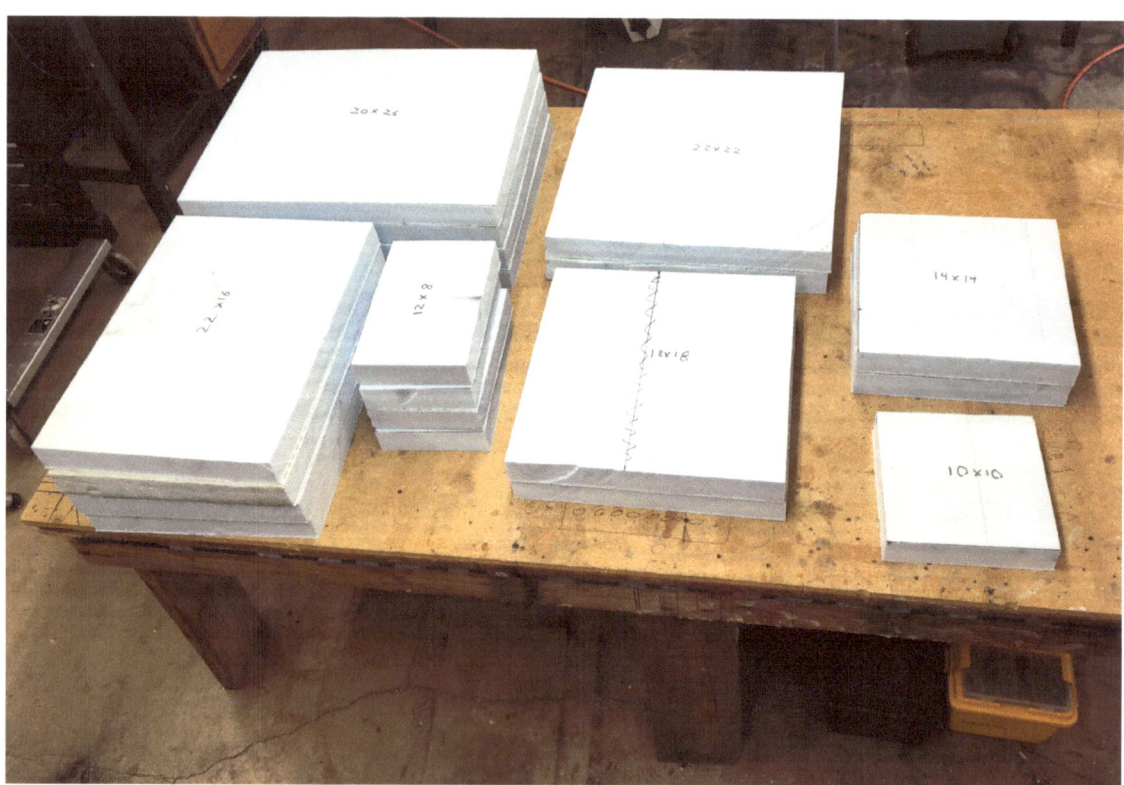

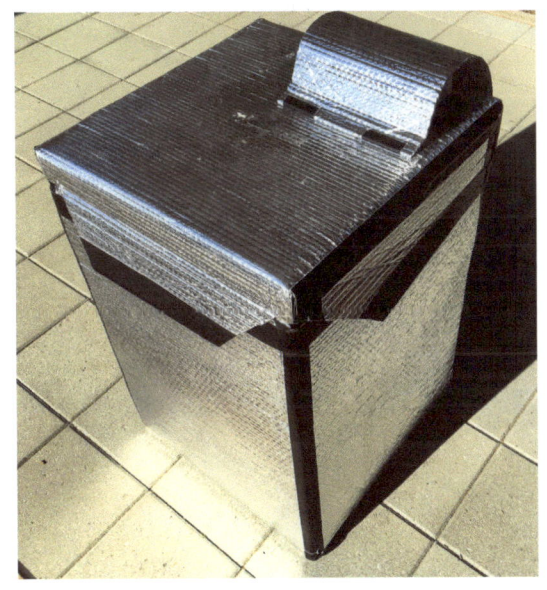

Step 3: Assemble the Cooler From Foam Sheets
The following steps detail how to assemble the complete cooler from sheets of foam and silver bubble wrap insulation. It is important to let the construction adhesive dry between a few different steps, so you should plan to spend 3 or so days to complete all of these steps.

Assembling the cooler from foam rectangles:

All parts cut from 2" (150mm) thick closed cell foam insulation. Parts glued with construction adhesive, and all cracks sealed with silicone caulk and/or aluminum furnace tape.

	Part #	Dimenstions (WxH)	Quantity
Lid	1	22 x 22 (559mm x 559mm)	2
	2	18 x 18 (457mm x 457mm)	2
Floor	3	14 x 14 (356mm x 356mm)	3
	4	10 x 10 (254mm x 254mm)	1
	5	20 x 26 (508mm x 660mm)	4
Body	6	16 x 22 (406mm x 559mm)	4
	7	12 x 8 (305mm x 203mm)	4

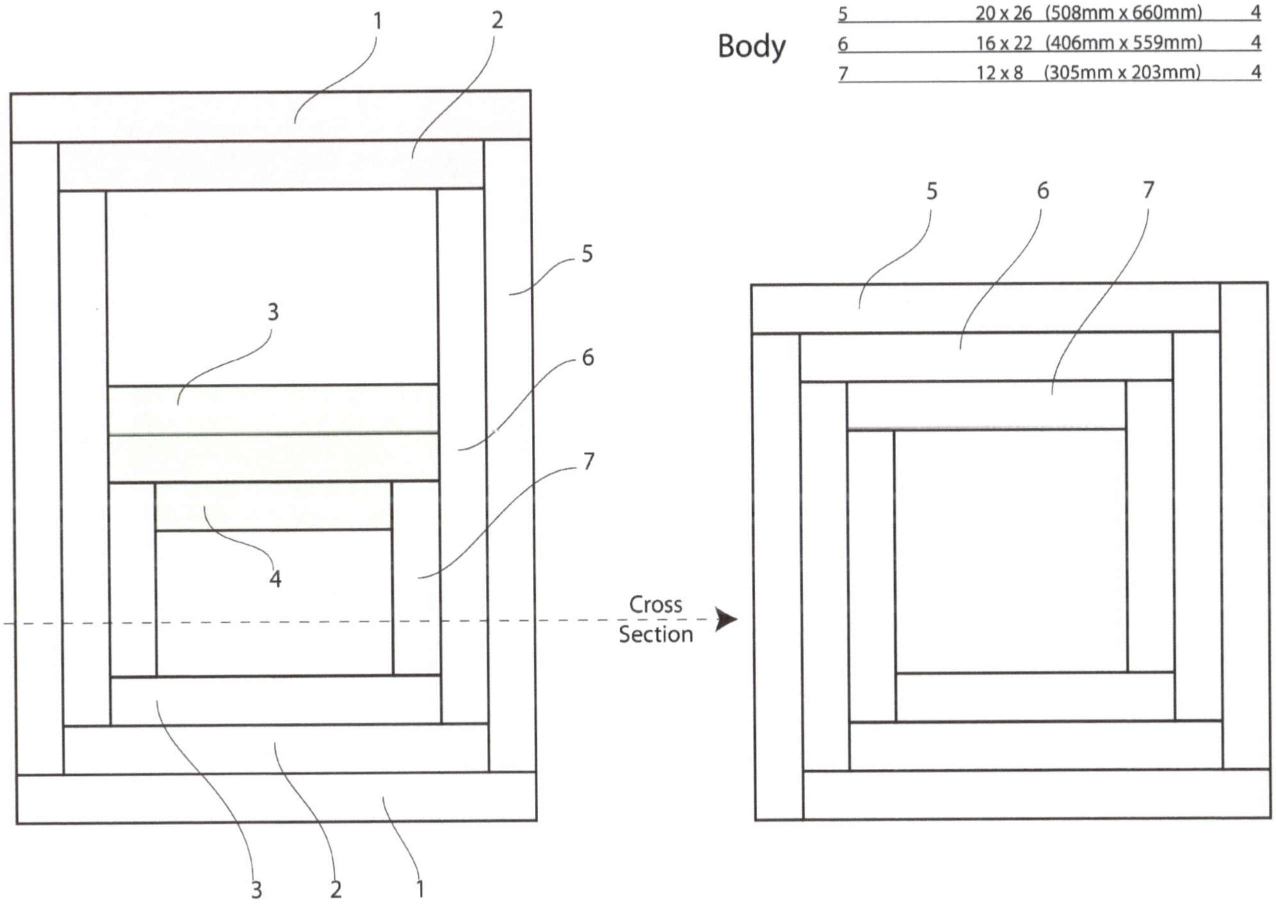

Cross Section →

2 x 14 in x 14 in
(356mm x 356mm)

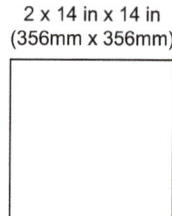

1 x 10 in x 10 in
(254mm x 254mm)

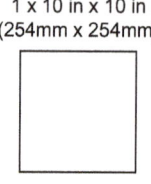

Construction
Adhesive

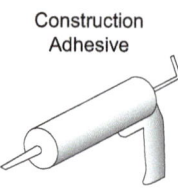

01. Build the cooler floor

Use construction adhesive to glue together the three squares cut for the cooler floor. Use a ruler to insure the smaller square is well centered.

Put a weight on top and set aside to dry for 24 hours.

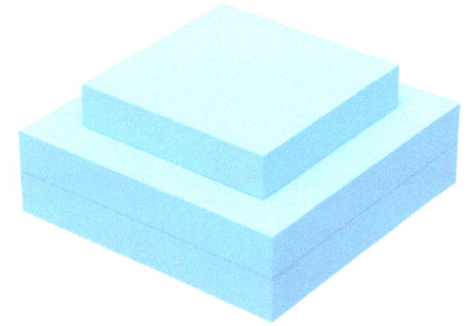

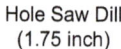

Aluminum
Tape

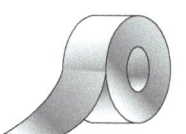

Hole Saw Dill
(1.75 inch)

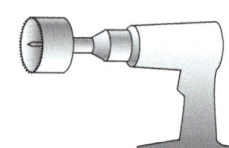

02. Finish the cooler floor

Cover the entire exterrior of the cooler floor with aluminum furnice tape. Be sure to smooth the tape sharply into the corners.

Use a 1.75 inch hole saw to cut two holes all the way through the cooler floor in the positions shown below:

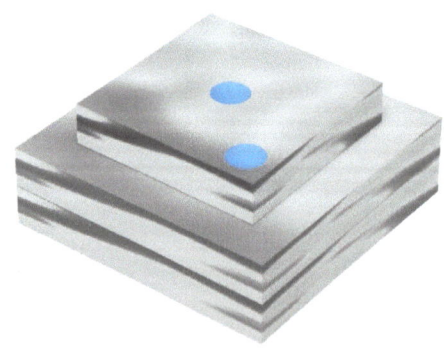

Position of holes:

Centered

3/4 in (2cm)

7

2 x 13 inch sections of PVC pipe
1.5 inch I.D. Sch.40

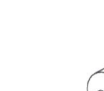

Construction
Adhesive

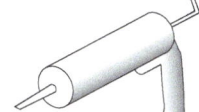

03. Put pipes through cooler floor

Cut two pieces of 1.5 inch (inner diameter) PVC pipe, measuring 13 inches long each.

Insert the PVC pipes through the full thickness of the cooler floor as shown below. Seal into place with construciton adhesive around the top and bottom edges of the pipes.

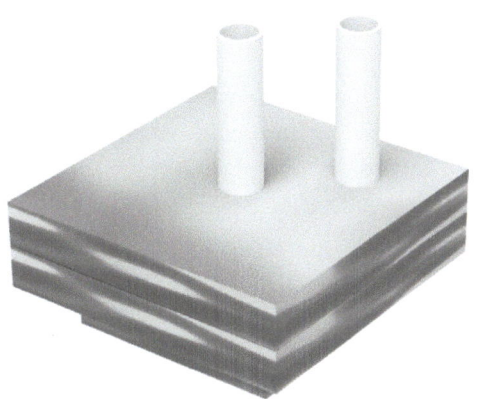

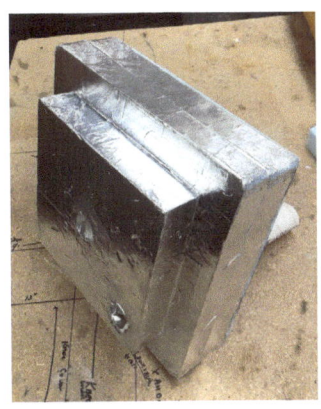

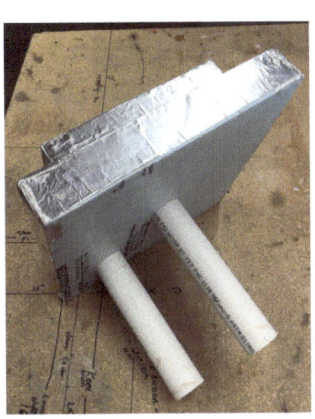

Mylar Bubble Insulation

Aluminum
Tape

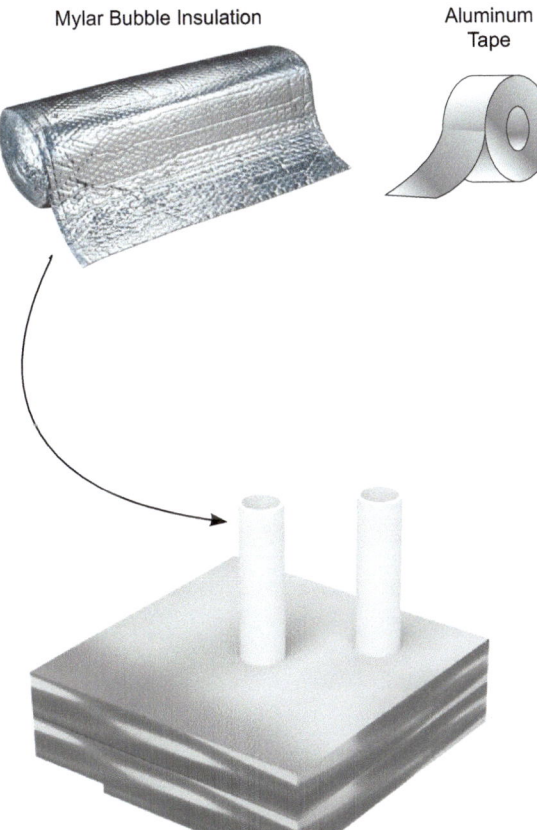

04. Insulate the cooler floor pipes

Insulate the pipes by wrapping them in three layers of mylar bubble furnace insulation. Insulation should not extend beyond the tops of the pipes.

Secure the insulation with aluminum tape. Seal around the bottom edges of the pipes with more tape.

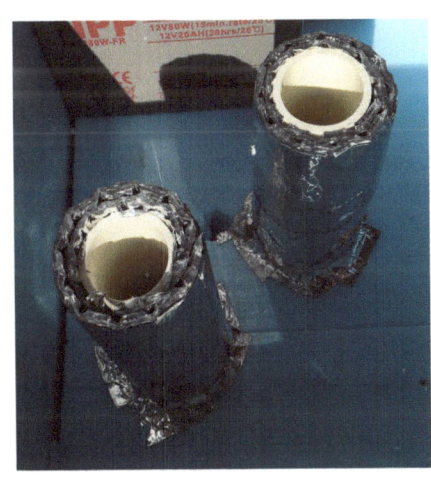

8

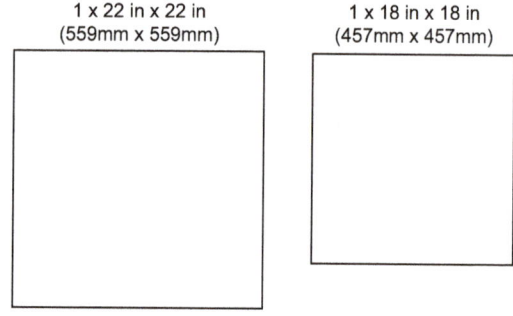

1 x 22 in x 22 in
(559mm x 559mm)

1 x 18 in x 18 in
(457mm x 457mm)

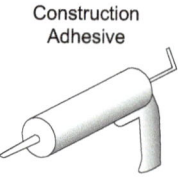

Construction
Adhesive

05. Construct the cooler lid

Use construction adhesive to glue one 18 x 18 inch square of foam to the top of one 22 x 22 inch square. Use a ruler to make sure the square is exactly centered and square in its placement.

Put a weight in the center and allow to dry overnight.

Aluminum
Tape

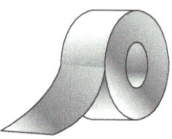

06. Finish the cooler lid

Cover the entire surface of the cooler lid with aluminum tape. It is OK to overlap the tape by a substantial amount to insure it sticks well and creates a smooth unbroken surface.

Be sure to push the tape all the way into the corners of the lid so they remain sharp 90 degree angles.

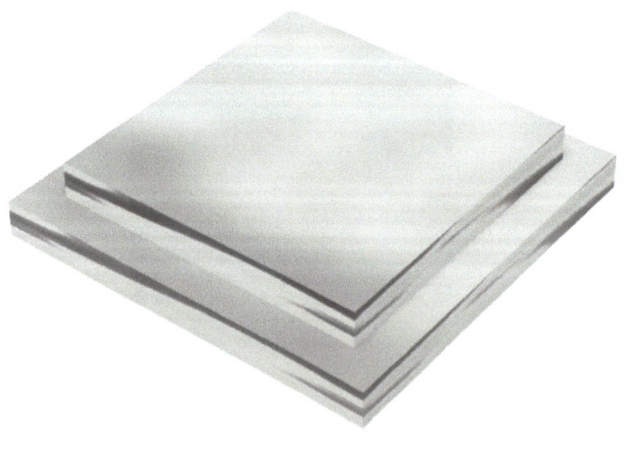

Create a Temperature Controlled Vaccine & Insulin Cooler

1 x 22 in x 22 in
(559mm x 559mm)

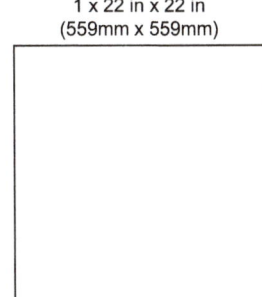

1 x 18 in x 18 in
(457mm x 457mm)

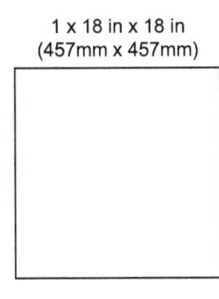

1 x 14 in x 14 in
(356mm x 356mm)

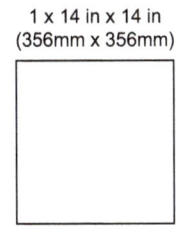

Construction
Adhesive

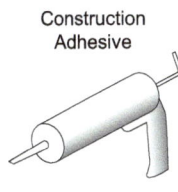

07. Construct the cooler base

Use construction adhesive to glue three squares of foam together: 14 x 14 inch ontop of the 18 x 18 inch on top of the 22 x 22 inch.

Be sure to center the squares carefully. Put a weight on the top and allow to dry overnight.

---

4 x 12 in x 8 in
(305mm x 203mm)

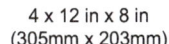
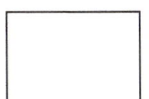

Construction
Adhesive

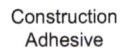
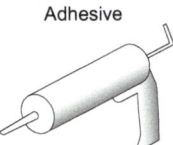

08. Construct the inner walls

Use construction adhesive to glue the edges of the inner walls into place as shown. Use aluminum tape as needed to hold in place.

Insert the cooler floor as a spacer. Be careful not glue the cooler floor!

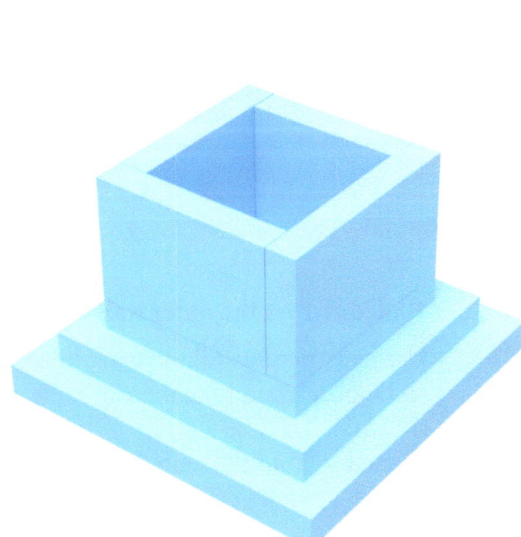

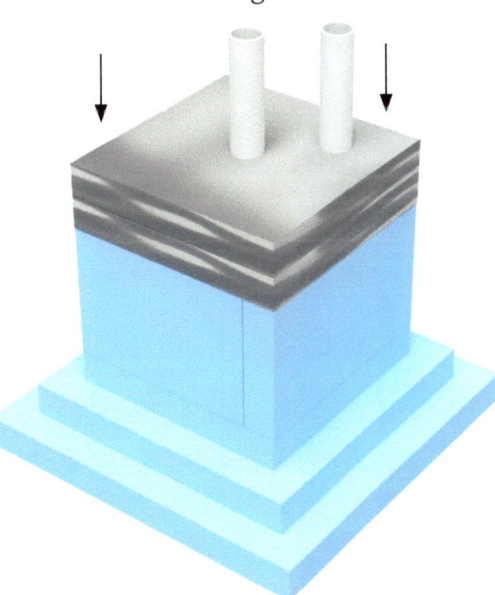

10

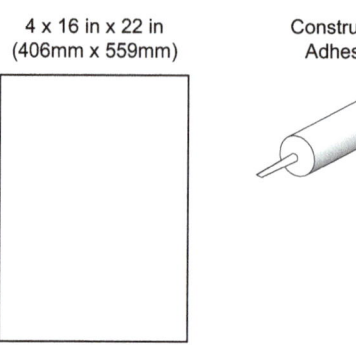

4 x 16 in x 22 in
(406mm x 559mm)

Construction
Adhesive

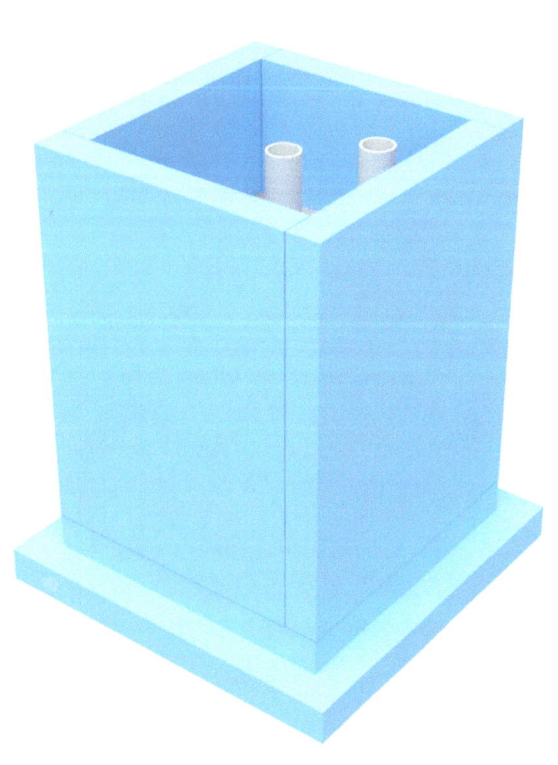

09. Construct the middle walls

Use construction adhesive to glue four rectangles around the inner walls as shown at left. Use aluminum tape as needed to hold the seams together to dry.

4 x 20 in x 26 in
(508mm x 660mm)

Construction
Adhesive

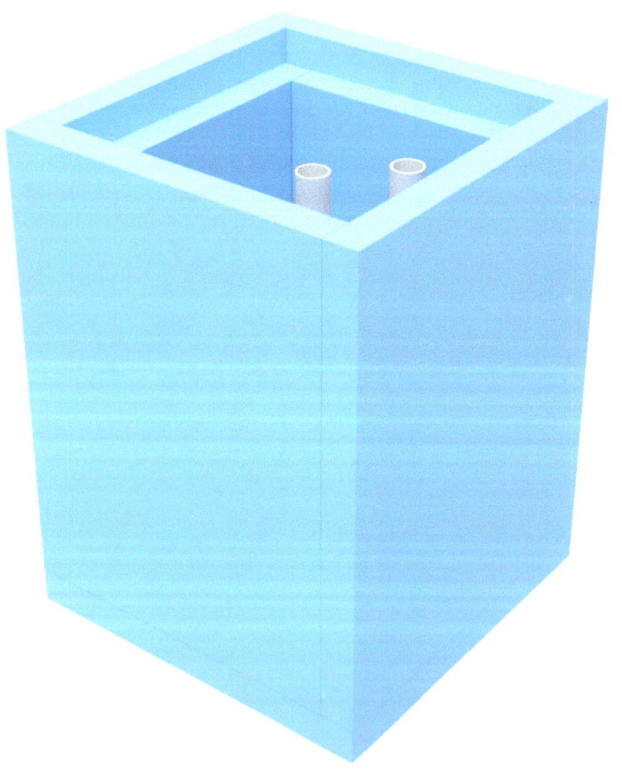

10. Construct the outer walls

Use construction adhesive to glue four rectangles around the middle walls as shown at left. Use aluminum tape as needed to hold the seams together to dry.

11

11. Insert the lid to hold the shape

Insert the completed lid into the top of the cooler as a spacer. This will insure a good fit for the lid once the adhesive is dry. Be careful not to glue the lid down!

Place weight on the top. Use straps and/or more aluminum tape to secure the outer walls. Allow to dry overnight.

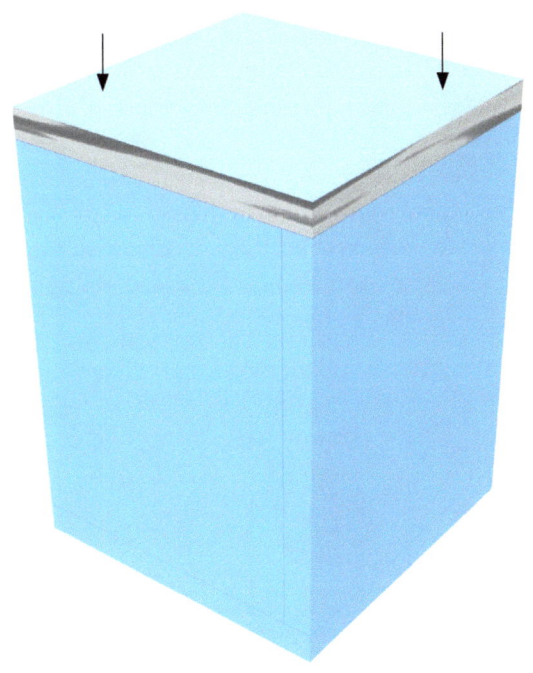

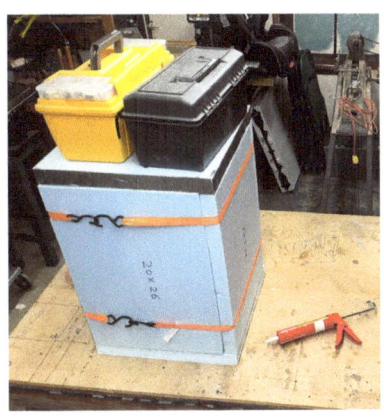

Silicone Caulk   Aluminum Tape

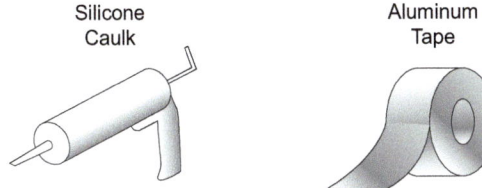

12. Seal the cooler with caulk

Once the construction adhesive has dried, use silicone caulk to seal all the inner   and outer seams of the cooler. Wear a glove and use your finger to wipe the caulk firmly down into all the seams so that the corners are sharp. Allow to dry overnight oncemore.

Once dry, use aluminum tape to structurally reinforce the cooler by taping over all of the outer seams.

The cooler floor should slide snuggly into place but be easily removable.

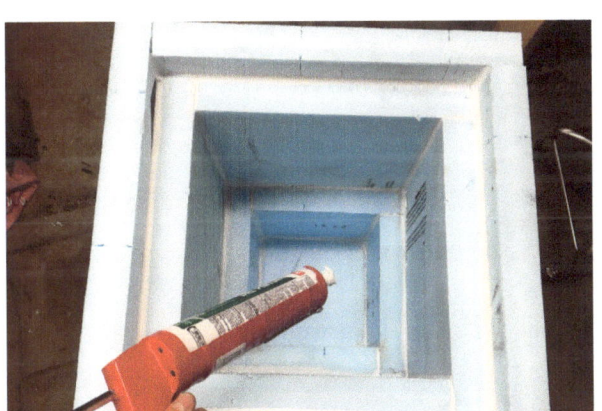

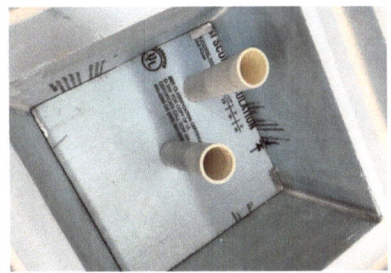

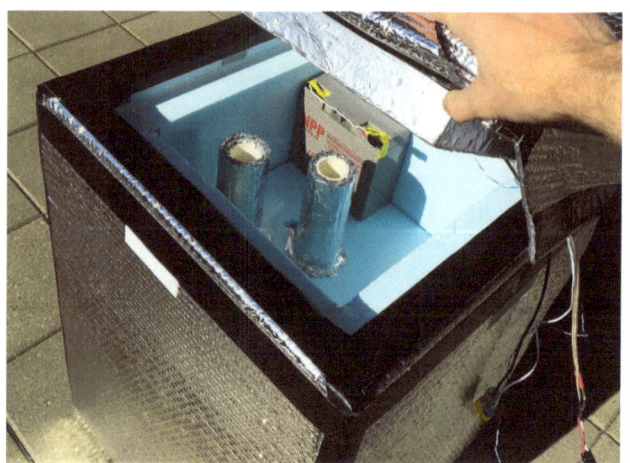

13. Cover with mylar insulation

Cut two lengths of mylar bubble insulation and snip the corners as shown below. Use high adhesion tape to cover the cooler body. First tape one piece to the cooler body, then tape the second piece to the first. Seal the vertical corners with more tape.

Seal around the top edge with tape to form a smooth padded seal for the lid to seat against.

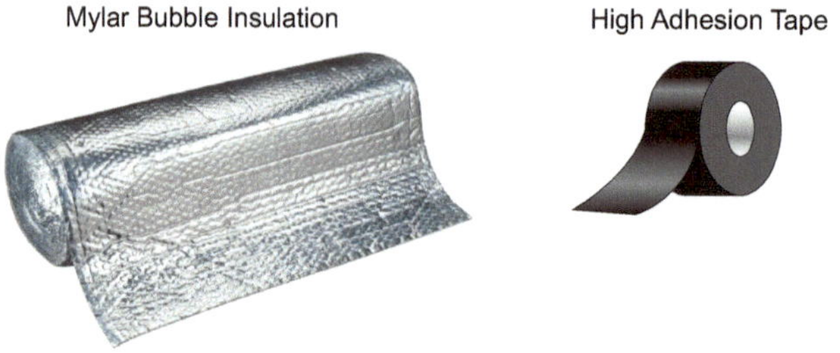

Mylar Bubble Insulation

High Adhesion Tape

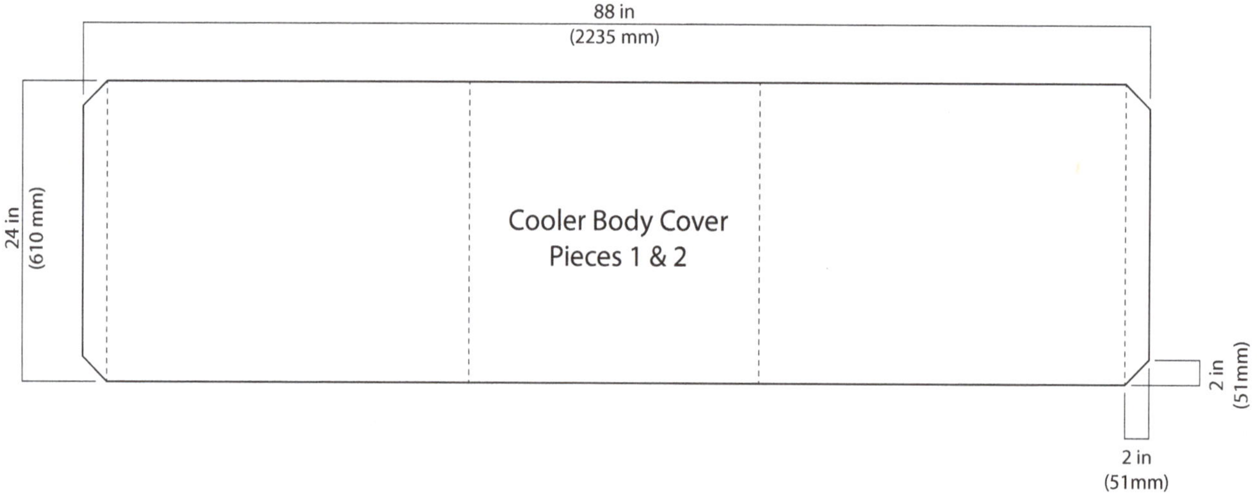

88 in
(2235 mm)

24 in
(610 mm)

Cooler Body Cover
Pieces 1 & 2

2 in
(51mm)

2 in
(51mm)

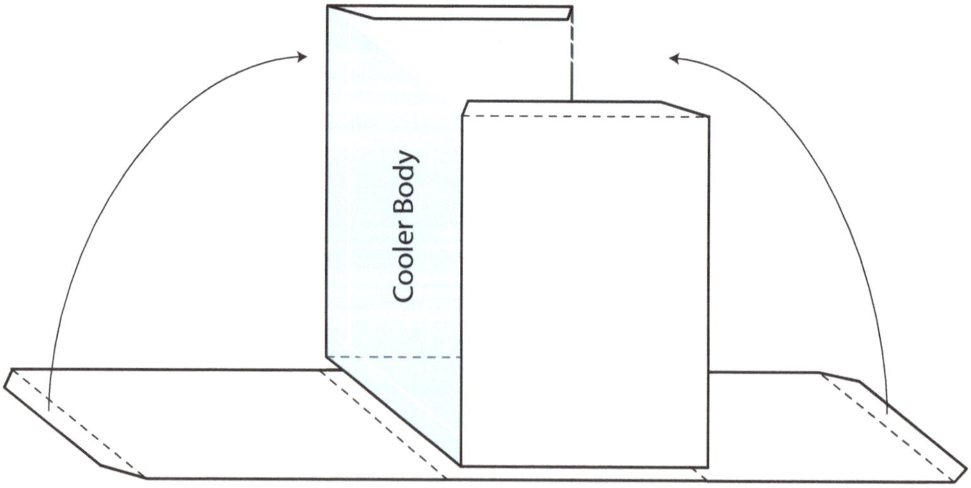

Cooler Body

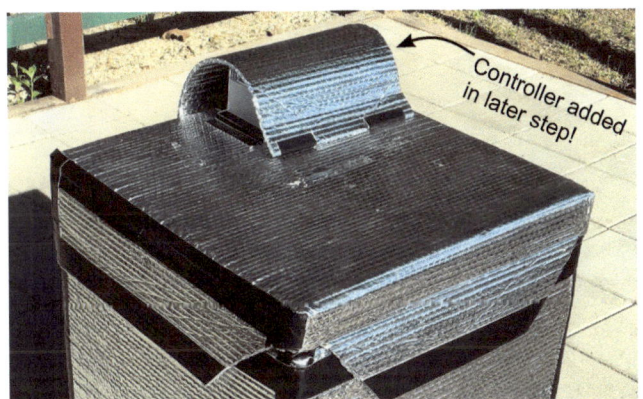

Controller added in later step!

14. Cover lid with mylar insulation

Cut out the pattern below for the lid. Fit the two pieces in place and tape to the lid from under the flaps. Put hook-and-loop strips under the flaps to hold the lid in place on the cooler.

Mylar Bubble Insulation

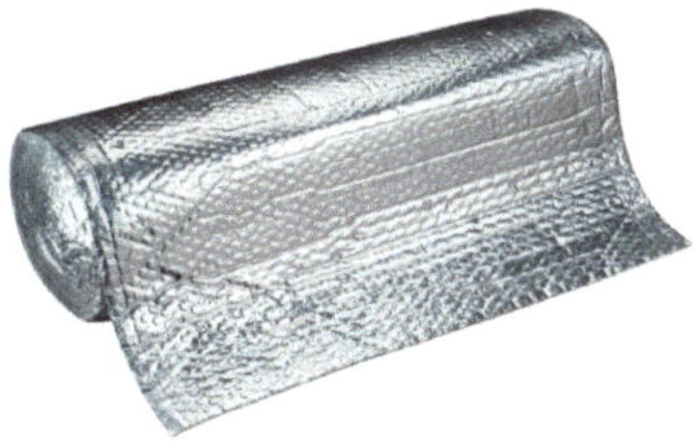

High Adhesion Tape

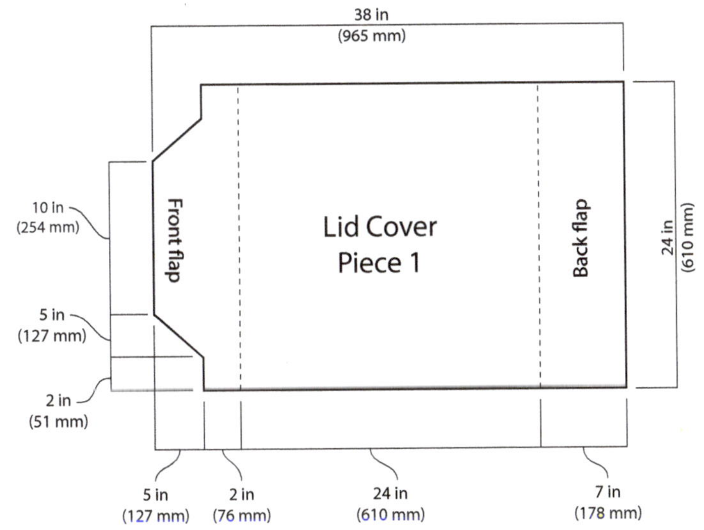

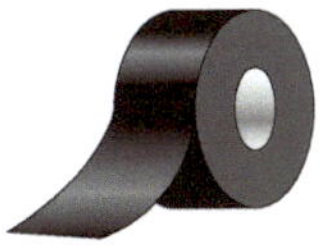

38 in
(965 mm)

10 in
(254 mm)

Front flap

Lid Cover
Piece 1

Back flap

24 in
(610 mm)

5 in
(127 mm)

2 in
(51 mm)

5 in
(127 mm)

2 in
(76 mm)

24 in
(610 mm)

7 in
(178 mm)

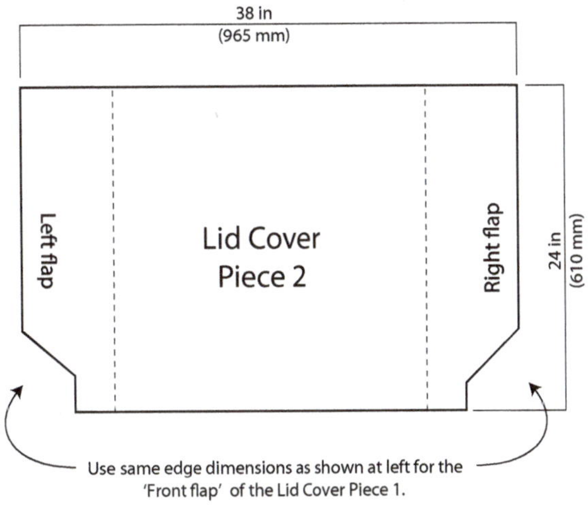

38 in
(965 mm)

Left flap

Lid Cover
Piece 2

Right flap

24 in
(610 mm)

Use same edge dimensions as shown at left for the 'Front flap' of the Lid Cover Piece 1.

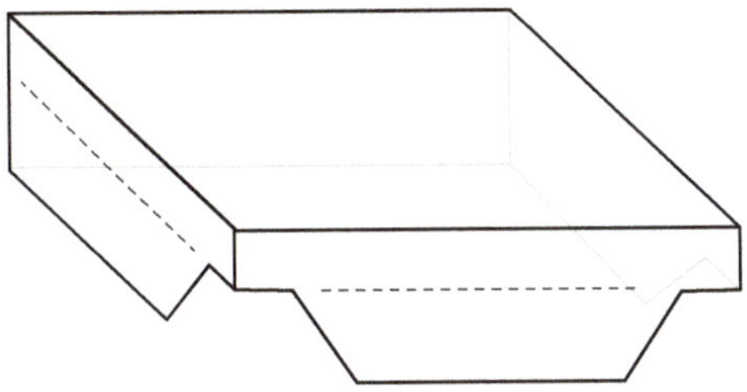

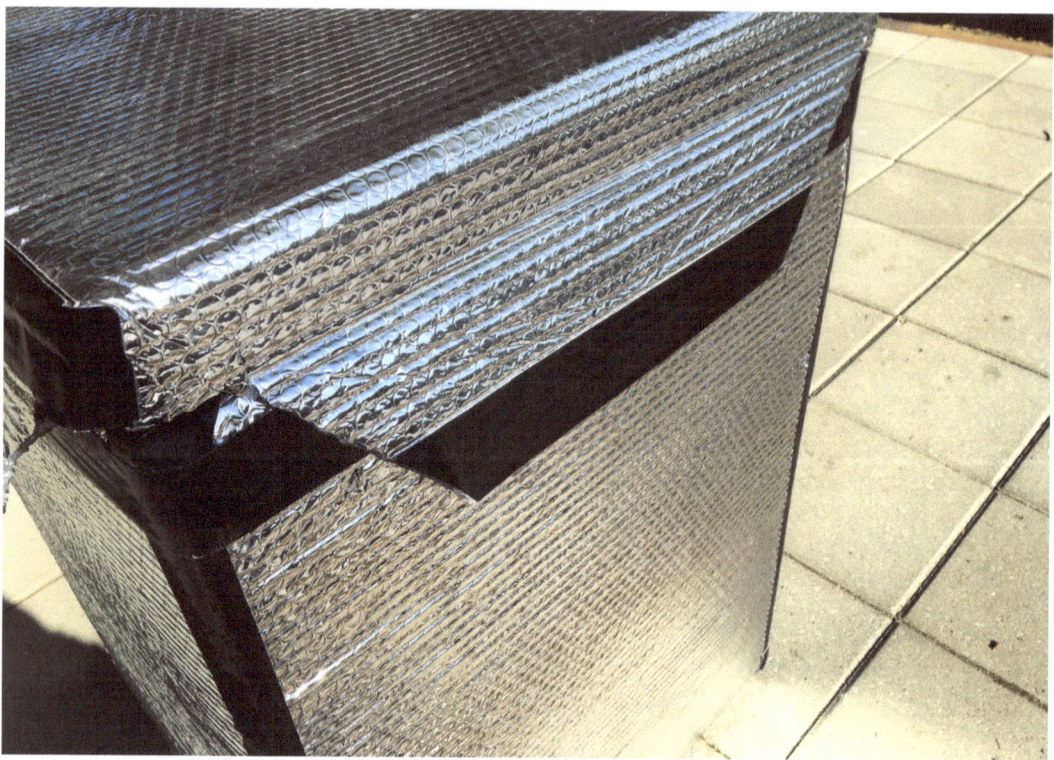

Detail of finished cooler box wrapped in silver mylar bubble wrap.

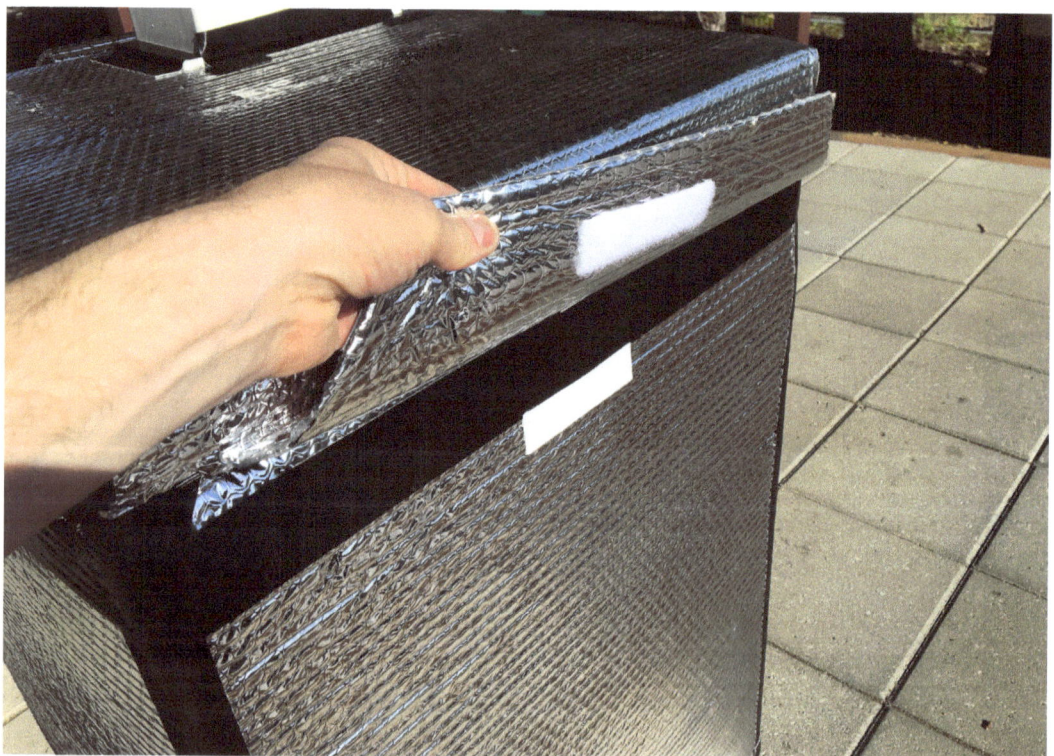

Top of cooler box is secured by hook and loop fasteners on each of four flaps.

Step 4: Assemble the Controller System

The following steps detail how to assemble the electronic components into a working Arduino based control system for the cooler.

Please refer to the list of parts below for the components needed to complete these steps. In some cases, there are very similar parts that can be used in place of the specific items listed.

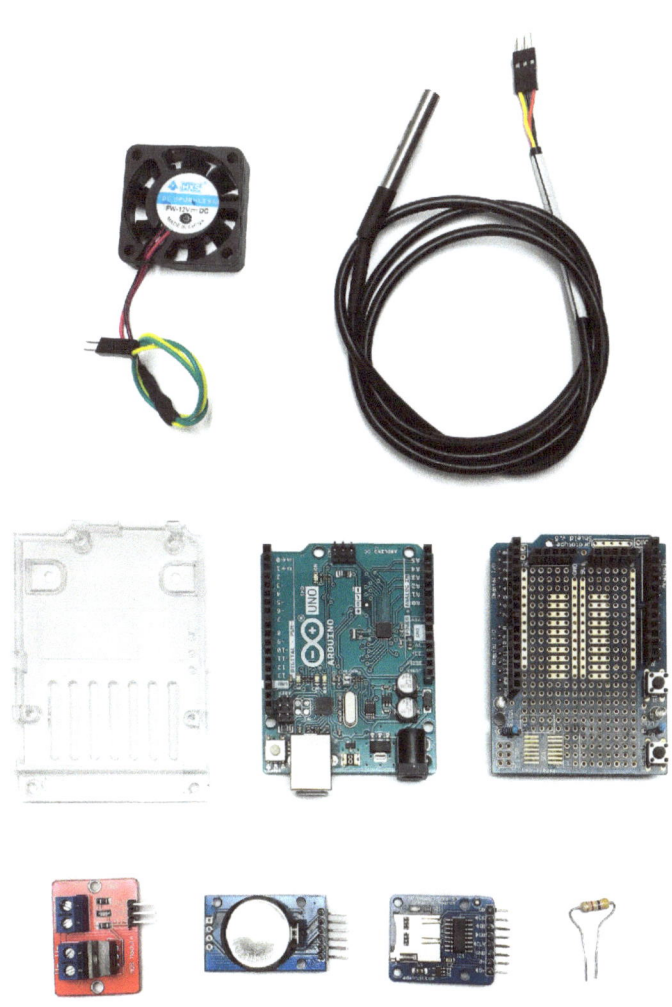

Electronic Parts for Thermostatic Control Box

MICROCONTROLLER: Arduino Uno microcontroller board or similar
PROTOTYPE BOARD: Alloet Mini breadboard prototype Shield V.5
MOSFET: IRF520 MOSFET driver module or similar
TEMPERATURE SENSORS: DFRobot DS18B20 waterproof digital sensor
12V SEALED LEAD ACID BATTERY: EXP12200 12 Volt 20 Ah or similar
12VDC PC FAN: 40mm x 10mm 12V cooling fan 0.12A
MICRO SD CARD READER: Adafruit ADA254
REALTIME CLOCK: DIYmore DS3231, based on DS1307 RTC
RTC BATTERY: LIR2032 coin cell
PLASTIC ENCLOSURE: Clear Cover ABS box, Size 7.9"x4.7"x2.94"
12 VOLT 3A FUSE: Automotive blade type fuse holder and fuse
CERTIFIED THERMOMETER: 'Thomas Traceable ' with vaccine bottle probe

Male Pin Headers

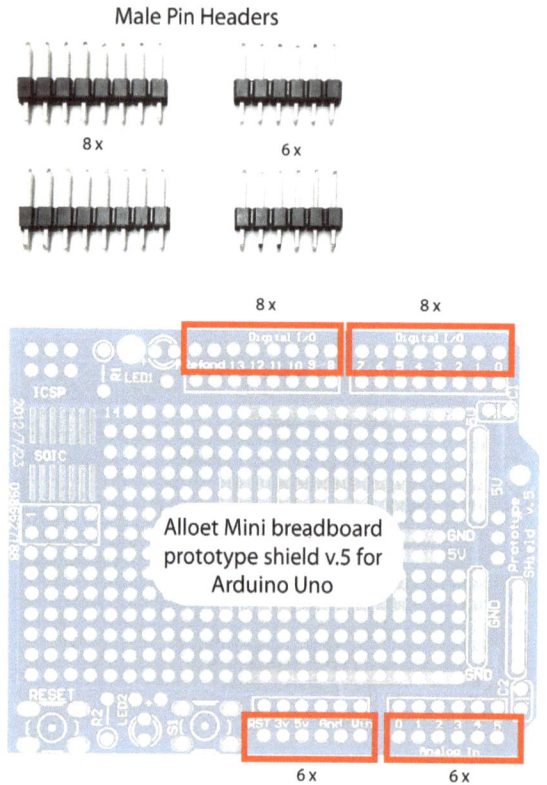

8 x

6 x

8 x

8 x

8 x

8 x

6 x

6 x

01. Pin Headers onto PCB

Use a soldering iron to solder a set of male pin headers to the underside of the prototype shield PCB in the locations shown at left.

These pin headers will allow the prototype shield to stack directly onto the top of an Arduino UNO by plugging into the UNO's female header sockets.

Female Pin Headers Sockets

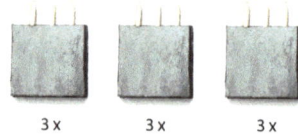

3 x

3 x

3 x

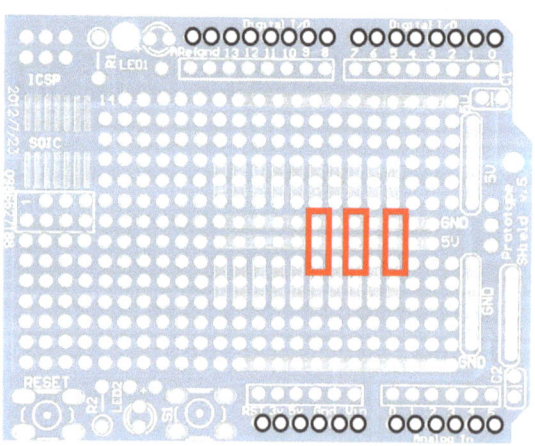

02. Pin sockets onto PCB

Use a soldering iron to solder a set female pin header sockets onto the PCB as shown at left. Notice how the sockets straddle the bus strips for GND and 5V.

These pin headers provide a place for the temperature sensors to connect to the board.

MOSFET Transistor Module

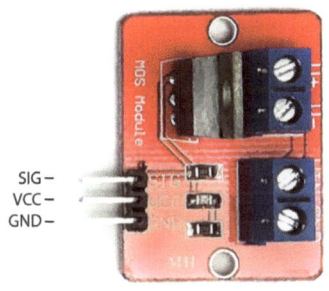

SIG —
VCC —
GND —

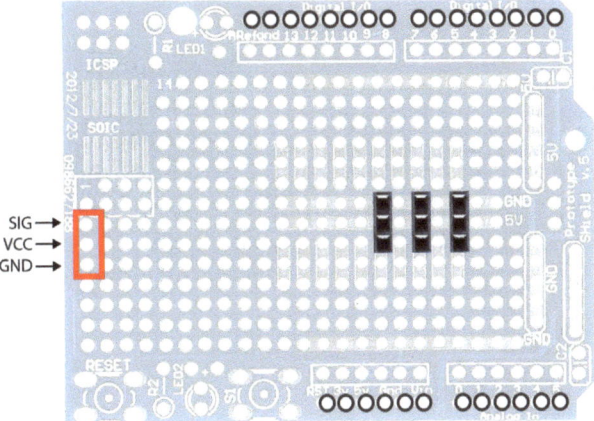

SIG →
VCC →
GND →

03. MOSFET board onto PCB

Use a soldering iron to solder the three pins of the MOSFET board onto the PCB as shown at left.

The MOSFET is a transistor switch that will allow the small power from the Arduino's output pins to control a 12 volt PC fan.

Real Time Clock Module

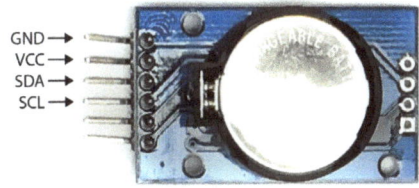

GND →
VCC →
SDA →
SCL →

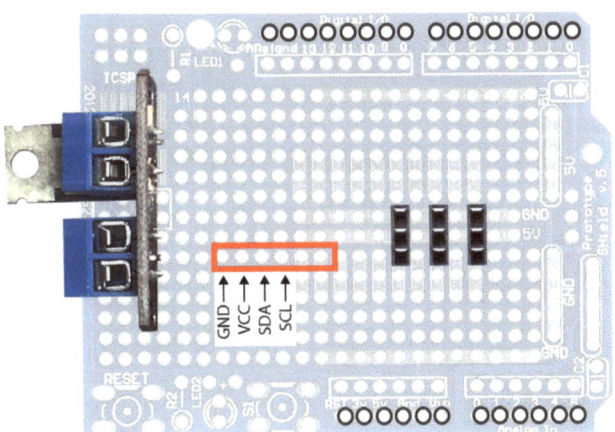

GND → VCC → SDA → SCL →

04. RTC module onto PCB

Use a soldering iron to solder the six pins of the Real Time Clock (RTC) onto the PCB in the positions shown at left.

The RTC has its own small battery so that it can hold the correct time and date even if the power is disconnected from the Arduino. It is useful for logging data because it lets you have an accurate time stamp.

18

Micro SD Card Module

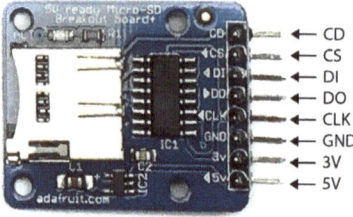

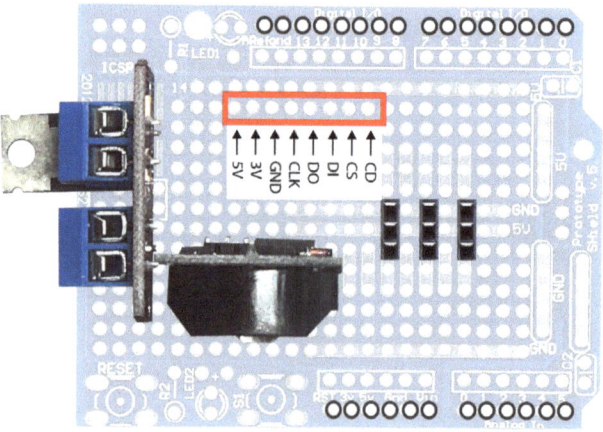

05. Micro SD card module

Use a soldering iron to solder the eight pins of Micro SD Card Module to the PCB in the location shown at left.

The Micro SD Card Module provides a stable memory location for storing recorded data from the temperature controller. This data can be useful for checking the performance of the cooler.

4.7K Resistor

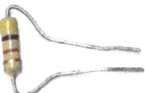

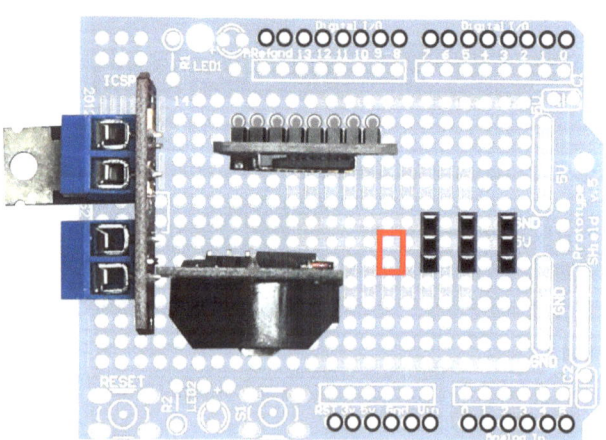

06. Put a resistor onto PCB

Use a soldering iron to solder a 4.7Kohm resistor onto the PCB as shown.

One of the resistor's wires connects to the 5V bus, while the other connects to all three of the bottom most poins of the female pin header sockets. This reistor is a 'pull-up' for the data line coming back from the temperatures sensors.

4 inch (10 cm) 26 gauge hook-up wires

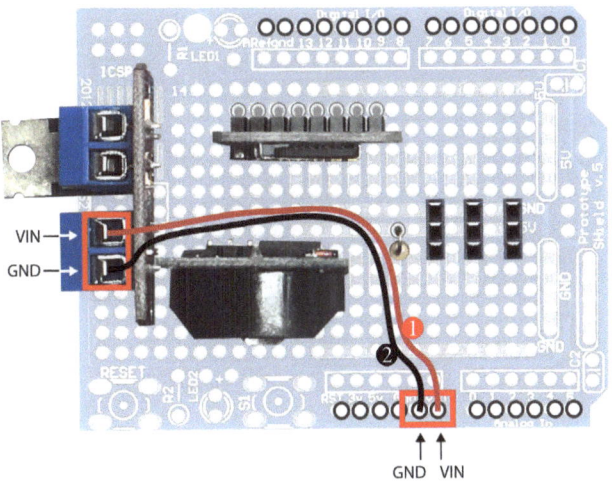

07. Conect power wires

Use a soldering iron to solder a pair of 26 gauge hook up wires onto the PCB as shown at left.

This pair of wires will provide power to the Arduino Module from the connected battery.

❶ The red wire connects to the PCB pin labeled VIN, and then to the VIN port in the MOSFET module.

❷ The black wire connects to the PCB pin labeled GND, and then to the GND port in the MOSFET module.

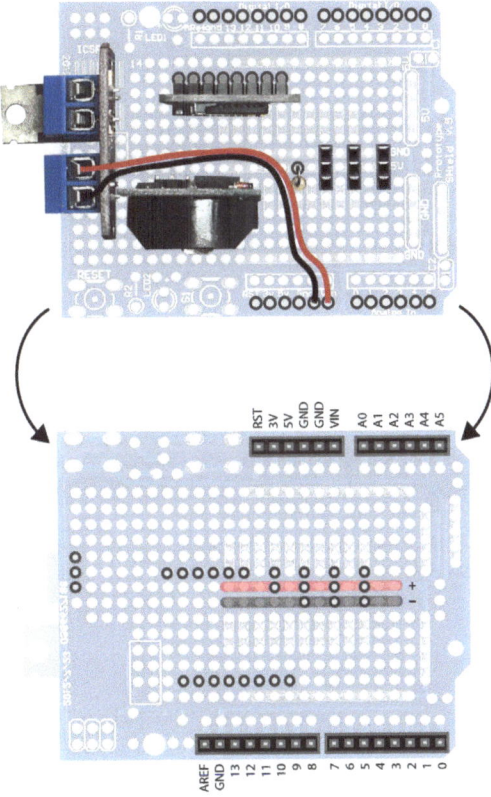

08. Flip the shield over

The next steps relate to attaching short lengths of wire between pins to complete the system. Use a soldering iron and a pair of wire strippers.

Looking at the bottom of the prototype shield, note the pin locations of the components and also the arduino header sockets (shown at left).

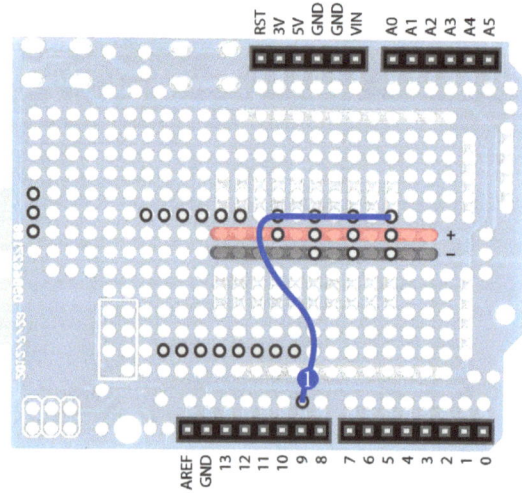

09. Temp. sensors bus wire

1 Use one wire to connect digital pin 9 to the resistor, and each of the three temperature sensor data bus pins.

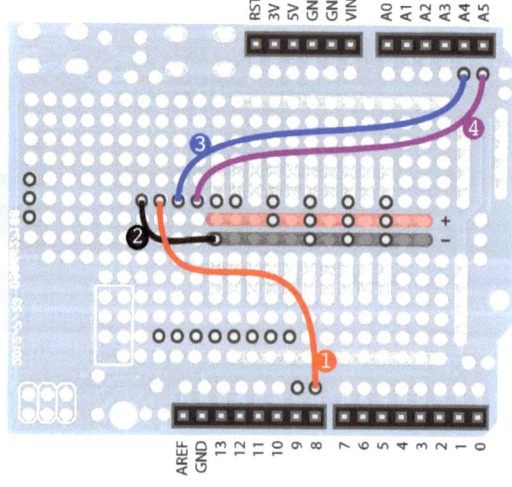

10. Real time clock wires

1 Connect the Arduino GPIO pin 8 to the clock VCC pin.

2 Connect the Arduino (-) bus to the clock GND pin.

3 Connect the Arduino pin A4 to the clock SDA pin.

4 Connect the Arduino pin A5 to the clock SCL pin.

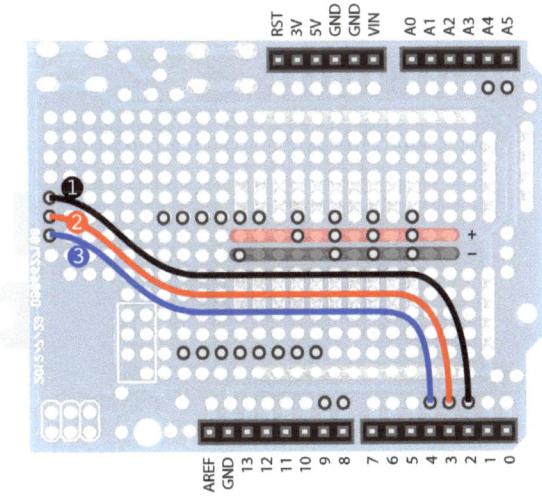

11. MOSFET board wires

❶ Connect the Arduino digital pin 2 to the transistor board GND pin.

❷ Connect the Arduino digital pin 3 to the transistor board VCC pin.

❸ Connect the Arduino digital pin 4 to the transistor board SIG pin.

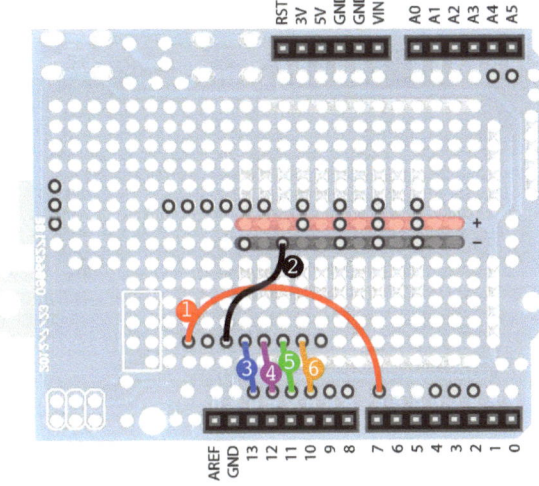

12. Micro SD board wires

❶ Connect the Arduino GPIO pin 7 to the Micro SD Breakout Board 5V pin.

❷ Connect the Arduino (-) bus to the Micro SD Breakout Board GND pin.

❸ Connect the Arduino digital pin 13 to the SD Breakout Board CLK pin.

❹ Connect the Arduino digital pin 12 to the SD Breakout Board DO pin.

❺ Connect the Arduino digital pin 11 to the SD Breakout Board DI pin.

❻ Connect the Arduino digital pin 10 to the SD Breakout Board CS pin.

22

Full schematic diagram of cooler control system

This schematic shows how the control system is wired internally, as well as how it connects to the external components such as the battery, sensor, and fan.

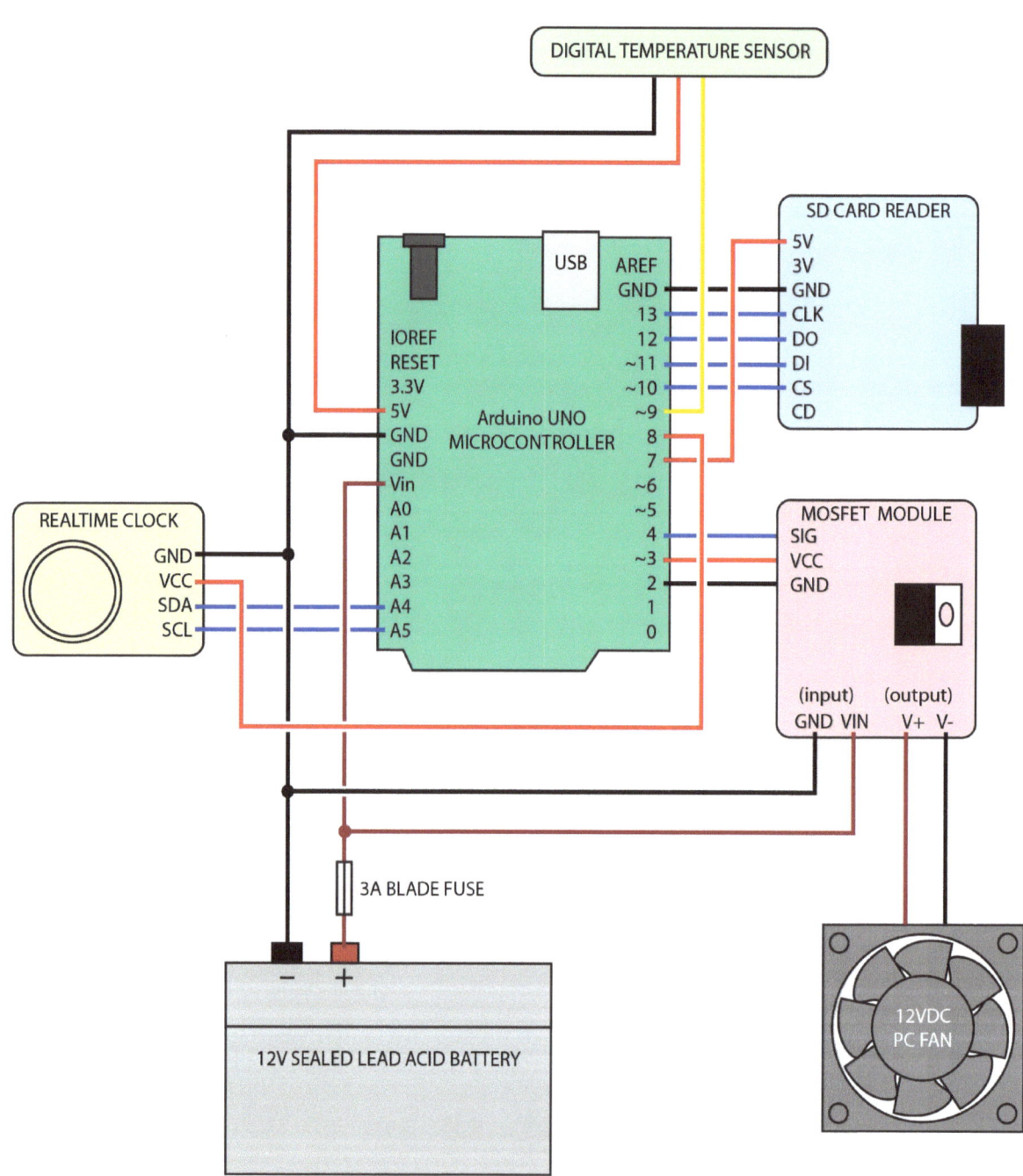

Step 5: Software Setup and Testing

First try this setup sketch

The setup sketch does two things. First, it lets you set the time and date in the Real Time Clock (RTC). Second, it tests all of the cooler controller's peripheral components and gives you a little report through the serial monitor.

Download the most current setup sketch here:
https://github.com/IdeaPropulsionSystems/ VaccineCoolerProject/tree/master/ CoolerSetupSketch_190503

Open the sketch in the Arduino IDE. Scroll down to the block of code commented as "Set the Time and Date Here." Fill in the current time and date. Now, double check that the following peripherals are setup and ready before you upload the sketch (see included electrical schematic image):

- Temperature Probe plugged into one of the 3 pin header sockets

- Micro SD card inserted into the reader module

- Coin cell battery inserted into the real time clock (RTC) module

- Hook up wires connected to the PC fan

- Fuse in the fuse holder of the battery wire.

- Arduino connected to the battery (being SURE it is not wired backward! + to VIN, - to GND!)

In the Arduino IDE, Select Arduino UNO from the list of boards, and upload. Once the upload is done, from the dropdown menu at the top, select Tools / Serial Monitor. This should display a little system report. Ideally, it should read something like this:

```
Cooler Setup Sketch - version 190504
START OF SYSTEM TEST ---------------------
TESTING REAL-TIME CLOCK: time[20:38]
date[1/6/2019]
TESTING TEMP. SENSOR: 22.25 C
TESTING SD CARD:
init done
Writing to dataLog.txt...dataLog.txt:
If you can read this, then your SD Card is
working!
TESTING FAN: Is the fan pulsing on and off?
END OF SYSTEM TEST ---------------------
```

Trouble-shoot the system

Usually for me, things never go quite as planned. Some system probably didn't work right. The setup sketch will hopefully provide a clue - the clock? The SD card? The most common problems with any microcontroller project usually have to do with one of these:

- Forgot to put a fuse into the battery wire, so no power?

- Forgot to put a micro SD card in the reader, so the system is hanging?

- Forgot to put a battery in the real time clock (RTC) so the system is hanging?

- Connected sensors are loose, disconnected, or connected in reverse?
- Wires for components are left disconnected, or connected to the wrong Arduino pin(s)?

- The wrong component is plugged into the wrong pins or is wired backward?

- There is a wire improperly attached that is shorting everything out?

Install the controller sketch

Once you have had a successful test with the CoolerSetupSketch, it's time to install the full controller sketch.

Download the most current controller sketch here:
https://github.com/IdeaPropulsionSystems/
VaccineCoolerProject

Just choose the CoolerThermostat.ino file with the most recent date. Connect the Arduino to your computer with a USB cable and upload the sketch with the Arduino IDE. You are now ready to physically install the whole system into the body of the cooler.

Step 6: Install the Arduino System

The following steps can be treated as a checklist or installing all the electronics. For the following steps, refer to the included photos of the finished project. Please refer to the diagram on the following page labeled "Open-Source Vaccine Cooler" while completing these steps.

1. Attach a pair of fan wires to the Arduino UNO module.

2. Attach a pair of 12-volt power wires to the Arduino UNO module.

3. Attach the DS18B20 temperature sensors to the Arduino UNO module. Just plug the sensor into one of the 3-pin socket(s) we installed in the prototype board. Pay attention to the wire colors, red goes to positive, black to negative, and yellow or white goes to the 3rd data pin.

4. Plug a USB printer cable into the Arduino's USB connector.

5. Use the 1.75" hole saw to drill a large round hole in the bottom of the electronics box.

6. Attach the Arduino UNO module to the bottom of the electronics box using self-adhesive hook-and-loop fastener strips.

7. Attach the calibrated vaccine thermometer to the underside of the clear lid of the box with hook-and-loop fastener strips. Connect its small liquid-buffered bottle probe wire.

8. Pass the following wires out of the box through the round hole in the bottom:
   - 12-volt power wires (12-18 gauge stranded copper 2 conductor speaker wire)
   - Arduino temperatures sensor(s) (DS18B20 with male 3 pin header connector on each)
   - USB printer cable (Type A Male to Type B Male)
   - Vaccine Thermometer probe (Included with calibrated thermometer)
   - Fan wires (twisted pair of stranded 26 gauge hook-up wire)

9. Open the lid of the cooler and use a knife or a drill to bore a 3/4 inch (2 cm) hole through the lid near one of the back corners. (See included pictures) Poke up through the mylar bubble wrap covering.

10. Feed all but the USB wire from the control box down through the lid from the top. Place the box onto the lid with the USB cable hanging out so it can be accessed later. Secure the box with high-adhesion tape.

11. Screw the clear lid of the electronics box onto the box.

12. Create a flap of additional silver mylar bubble wrap insulation to cover the box and protect it from direct sunlight. (See included pictures.)

13. Inside the cooler, place the 12 volt 20AH battery near the back of the compartment. The battery will remain inside the chamber alongside the cargo. It will work well even at 5°C, and will serve as some thermal buffering, similar to a water bottle.

14. Attach both of the temperature probes (the thermometer's bottle probe and the Arduino probe) to the base of the center pipe using high-adhesive tape.

15. Inside the cooler, use aluminum tape to attach the fan so that it blows down into the corner pipe. Connect its wires to the wires from the controller. The fan blows down the corner pipe, and super chilled will fountain up into the cargo chamber from the center pipe.

Open-Source Vaccine Cooler

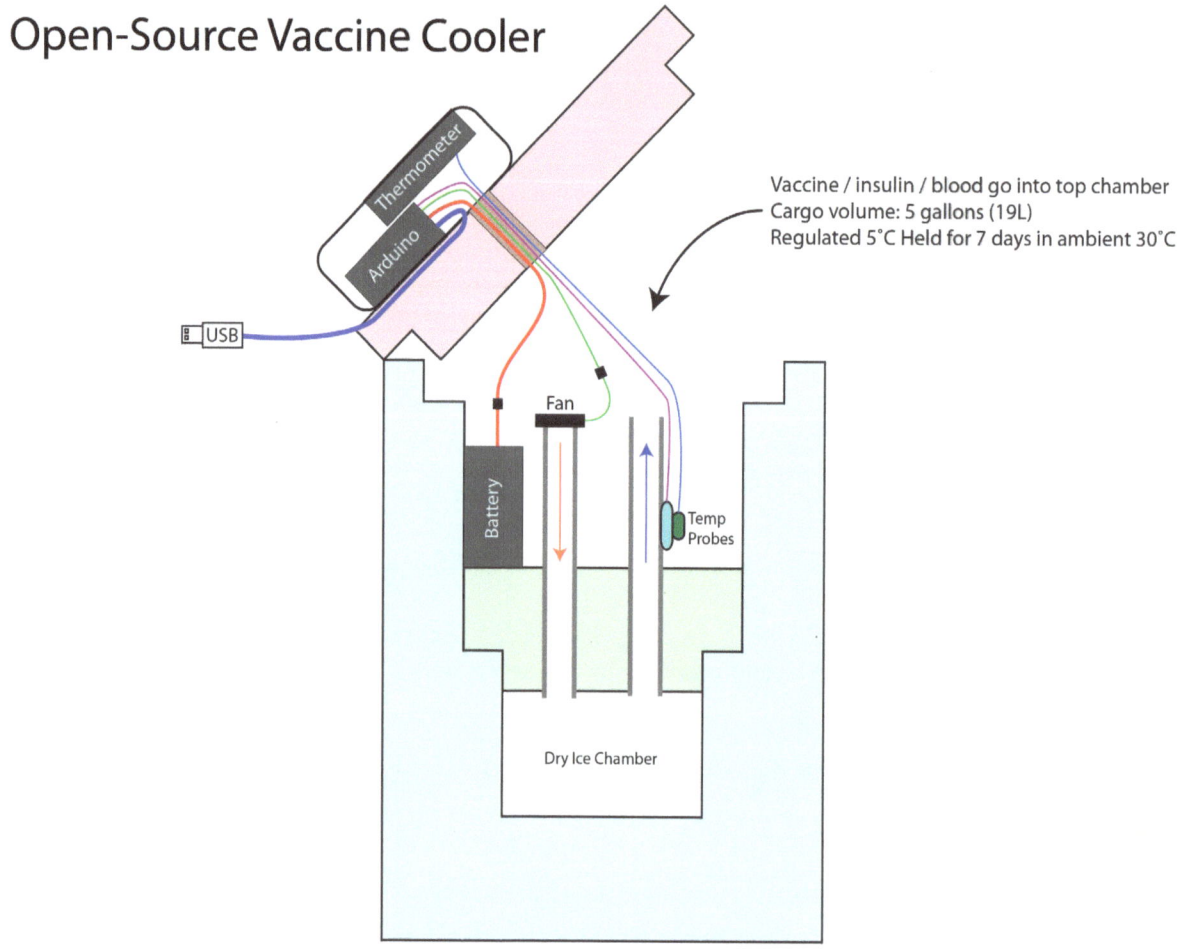

Vaccine / insulin / blood go into top chamber
Cargo volume: 5 gallons (19L)
Regulated 5°C Held for 7 days in ambient 30°C

Vaccine cooler with all subsystems connected. Note the location of the battery, fan, and temperature probes. All wires feed up into the Arduino box.

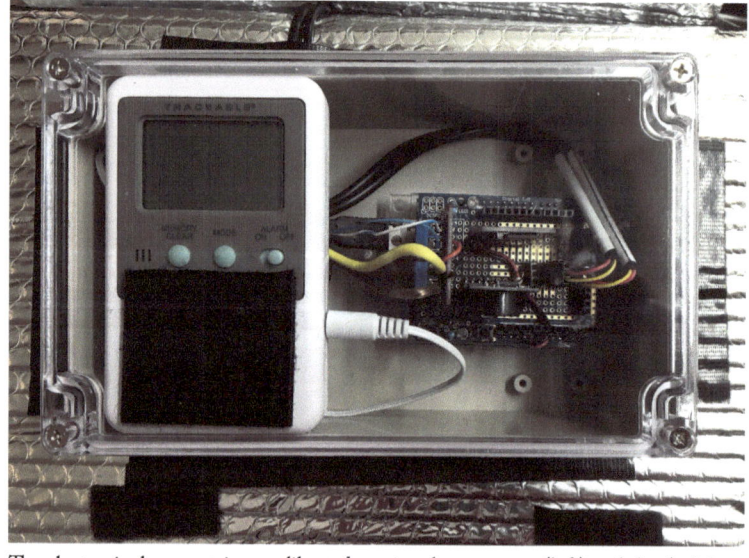

The electronics box contains a calibrated vaccine thermometer (left) and the Arduino UNO with custom shield (right). All wires feed down through bottom of box and through the cooler's lid.

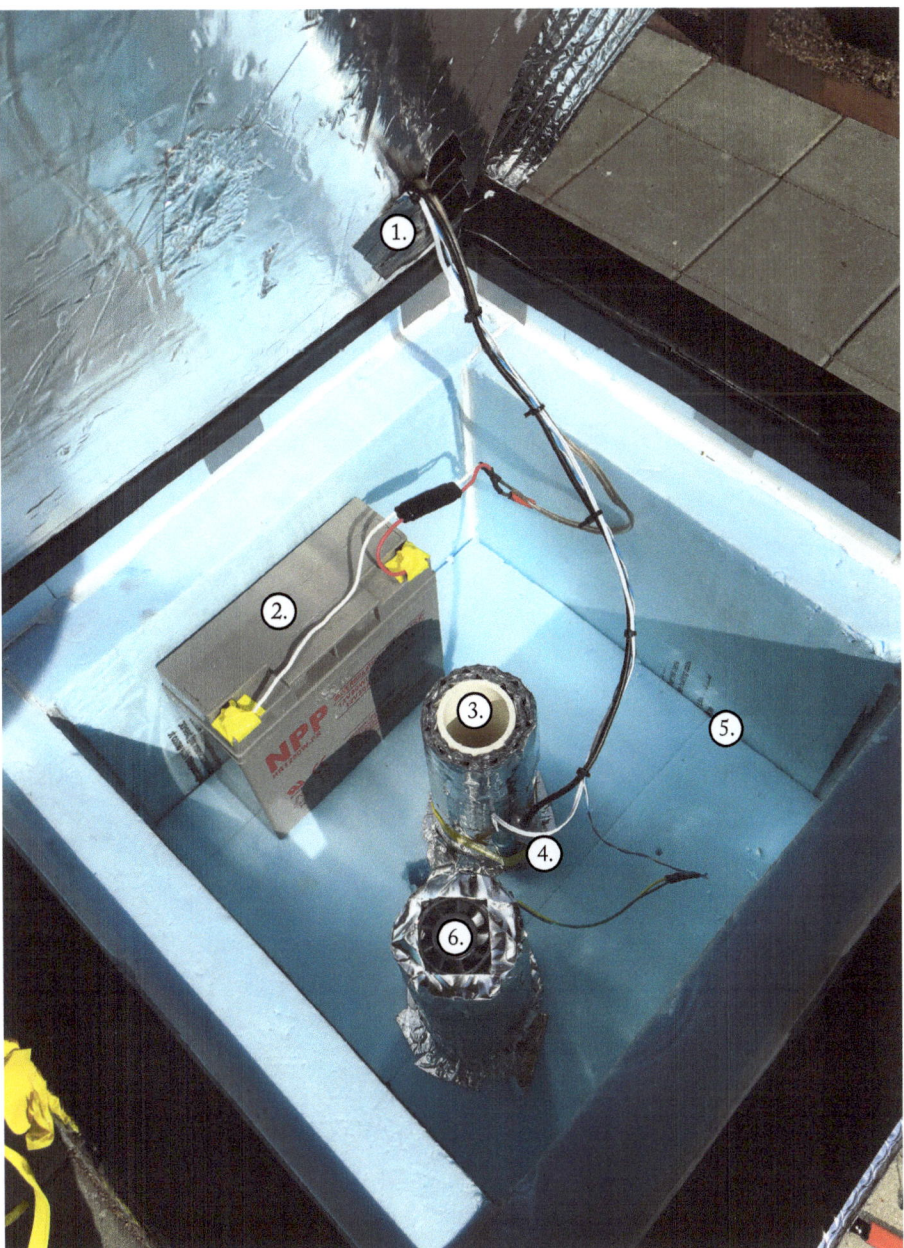

1. Cables from the controller are firmly held in place with high-adhesion tape. The hole is taped over to hold in cool air.

2. Sealed 12 volt battery lives in the cooler chamber. It works just fine at 5C and helps to buffer the temperature of the cargo. Tape the battery in place with high adhesion tape during use.

3. Super chilled air from the ice chamber fountains out of the top of this pipe when the fan is running.

4. Temperature sensors from the vaccine thermometer and from the thermostat are buffered in small water bottles and taped near the bottom of the insulated center pipe.

5. Use aluminum tape to seal around the cooler floor when in operation. The seal lets the ice last longer.

6. The fan blows the cargo chamber's air down into the ice chamber for a few seconds at a time according to the thermostat.

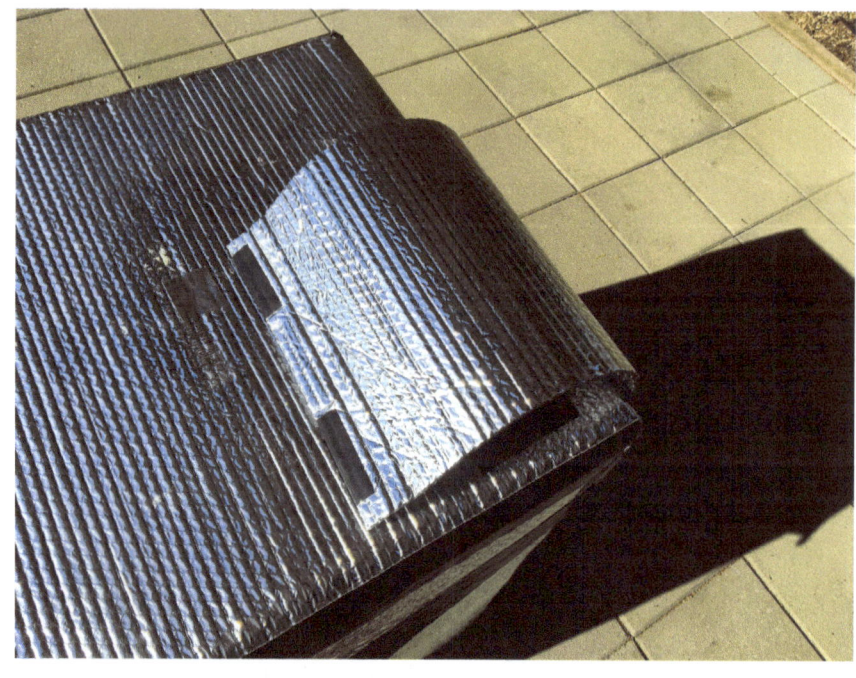

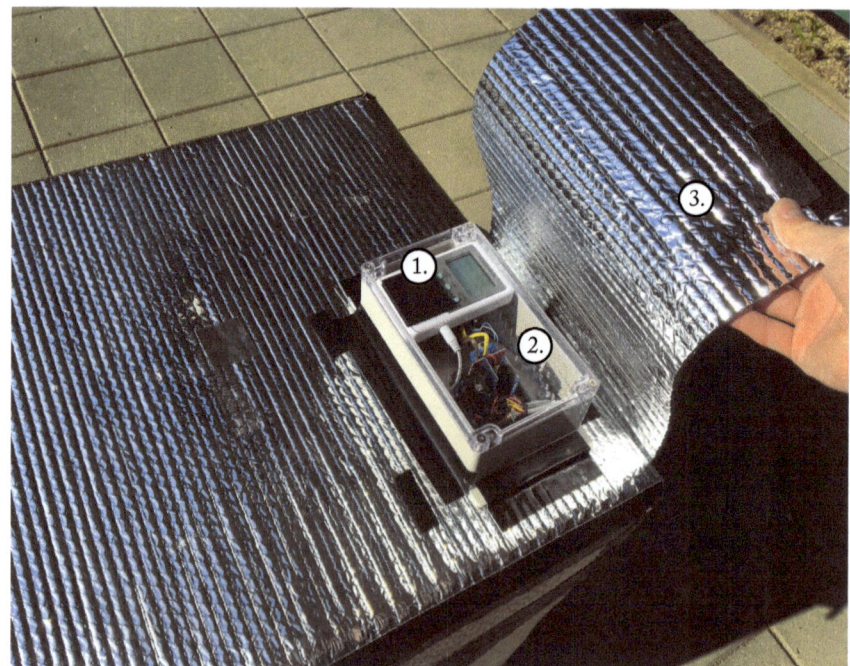

1. Certified calibrated vaccine thermometer is held to inside of clear lid by hook & loop strips.

2. Arduino controller is kept safe from dirt and dust inside case. It controls the temperature of the cooler and maintains a log of temperature over time.

3. Protective flap of silver bubble insulation

Step 7: Cooler Startup and Operation

1. Format the Micro SD card - the temperature will be logged to this chip

2. Recharge the 12 volt battery

3. Purchase a 25 lb (11.34kg) block of dry ice, cut to dimensions 8 in x 8 in x 5 in (20 cm x 20 cm x 13 cm).

4. Install the ice block by first placing the block flat on towel on a table. Slide the silver Mylar liner over the block so that only the bottom surface is exposed. Now lift the entire block, flip over so the bare ice faces upward, and slide the whole block into the dry ice chamber below the cooler floor.

5. Replace the cooler floor. Use aluminum tape to tape around the outer edge of the floor.

6. Place the 12 volt battery into the body of the cooler. You may wish to secure it to the cooler wall with strips of high adhesive tape.

7. Connect the controller power wire to the battery.

8. Check to see that the temperatures probes are securely taped.

9. Load water bottles into the cargo compartment to fill nearly all of the space. These will buffer the temperature.

10. Set the cooler somewhere out of direct sunlight and allow 3-5 hours for the temperature to stabilize at 5C.

11. Once the temperatures has stabilized, temperature sensitive items may be added by removing water bottles and filling that volume with cargo.

12. This cooler with a fresh charge of ice and power will sustain a controlled 5C for up to 10 days without any additional power or ice. The performance is better if the cooler is kept out of direct sunlight. The cooler can be moved and is resistant to shock in most respects; it should, however, be kept upright. If tipped over, simply stand it back up, no harm done.

13. The remaining electrical power in the battery can be measured directly with a small volt meter. The system requires a minimum of 9 volts to function properly.

14. The remaining ice can be measured directly with a metal tape measure by measuring down the center pipe-hole up to the top edge of the PVC pipe. See the attached table for measurements to remaining ice-weight.

15. Temperature logging data can be downloaded by attaching the USB wire to a laptop running the Arduino IDE. Connect, and open the Serial Monitor. The Arduino will automatically restart and read the full log out through the serial monitor. The cooler will continue to function without interruption.

16. The data can be downloaded from the enclosed MicroSD Card, but the system *must be powered-down before pulling out the tiny chip.*

The following pages include photos that show some details related to setting up and operating the cooler. Always wear gloves when handling dry ice. Be certain the cooler is set up and in a well ventilated area.

Create a Temperature Controlled Vaccine & Insulin Cooler

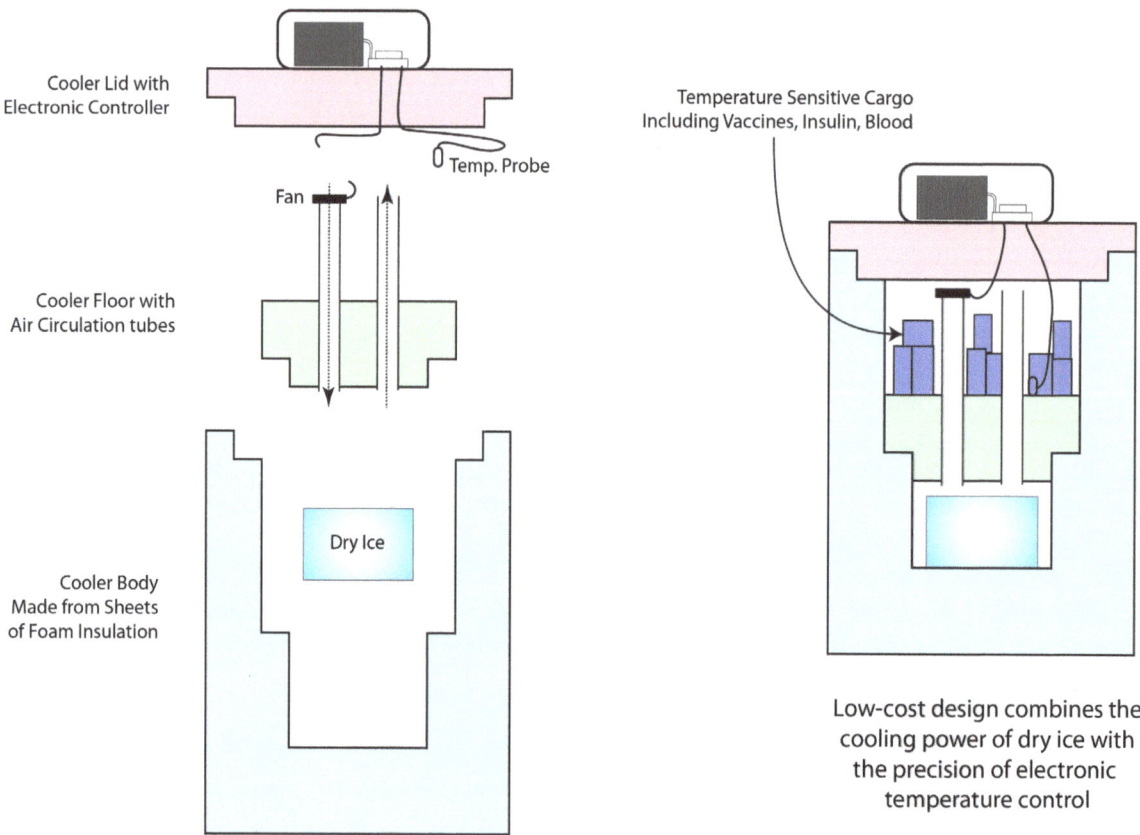

Cooler Lid with Electronic Controller

Temp. Probe

Fan

Cooler Floor with Air Circulation tubes

Cooler Body Made from Sheets of Foam Insulation

Dry Ice

Temperature Sensitive Cargo Including Vaccines, Insulin, Blood

Low-cost design combines the cooling power of dry ice with the precision of electronic temperature control

This diagram shows how the lid, floor, and body of the cooler are assembled for operation.

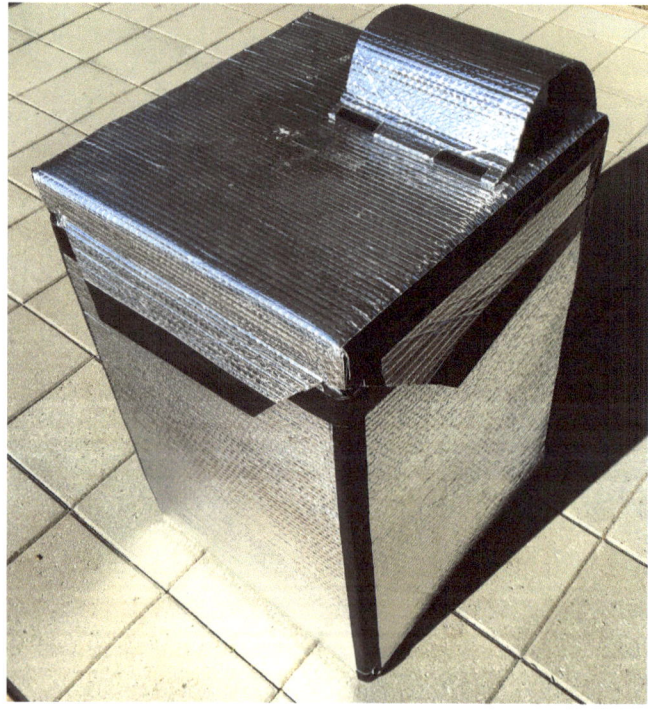

The fully assembled cooler, sealed and protected from direct sunlight by silver bubble wrap insulation.

Create a Temperature Controlled Vaccine & Insulin Cooler

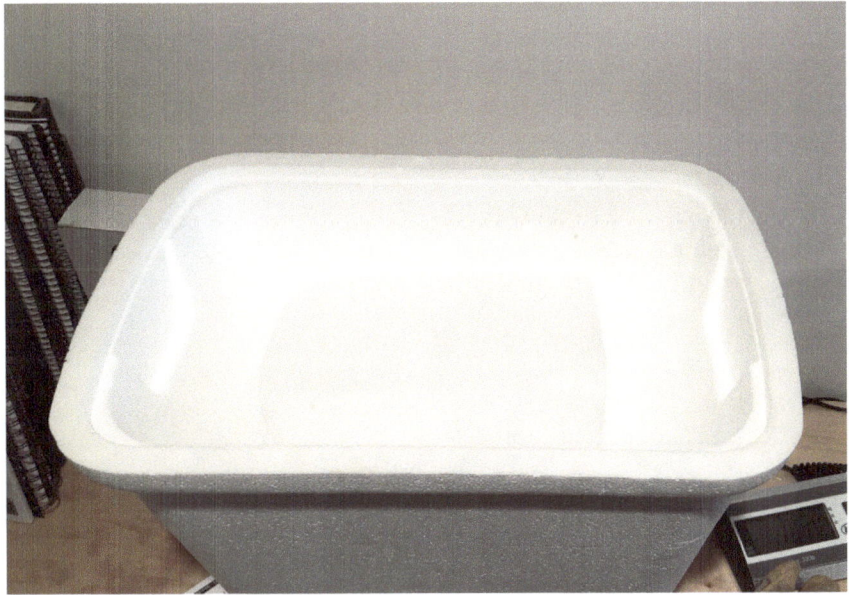

Dry ice is **EXTREMELY** cold and can burn your hands. Always wear gloves when handling. Also be sure to use in a well ventilated area. Do not leave a large chunk of dry ice like this in your car with the windows closed!

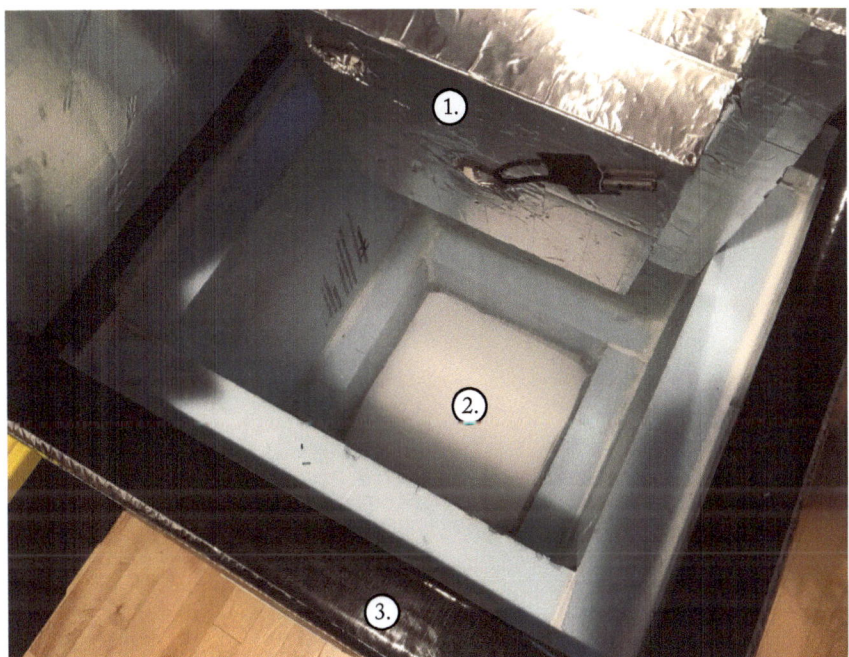

1. Cooler floor pulled up to install dry ice.

2. Block of 25 pounds (11.34 kg) of dry ice in insulation

3. Soft padded lid seal all the way around the top edge of cooler. It is created with tape over the exterrior bubble wrap insulation.

Step 8: Notes and Data

This cooler was designed to be a decent balance of size, weight, capacity, and cooling-time. The exact dimensions described in the plans can be considered a default starting point. They can be modified to better suit your needs. If, for instance, you require a longer cooling time, the dry-ice chamber can be constructed with a taller volume for more ice. Likewise, the cargo chamber can be built wider or taller. Care should be taken to experimentally prove-out any design changes you make, however. Small changes can have a large impact on overall system performance.

A set of recorded data from experiments can be downloaded from the online repository GitHub from the following location:

Download experimental data:
https://github.com/IdeaPropulsionSystems/
VaccineCoolerProject/tree/master/Experimental_Data

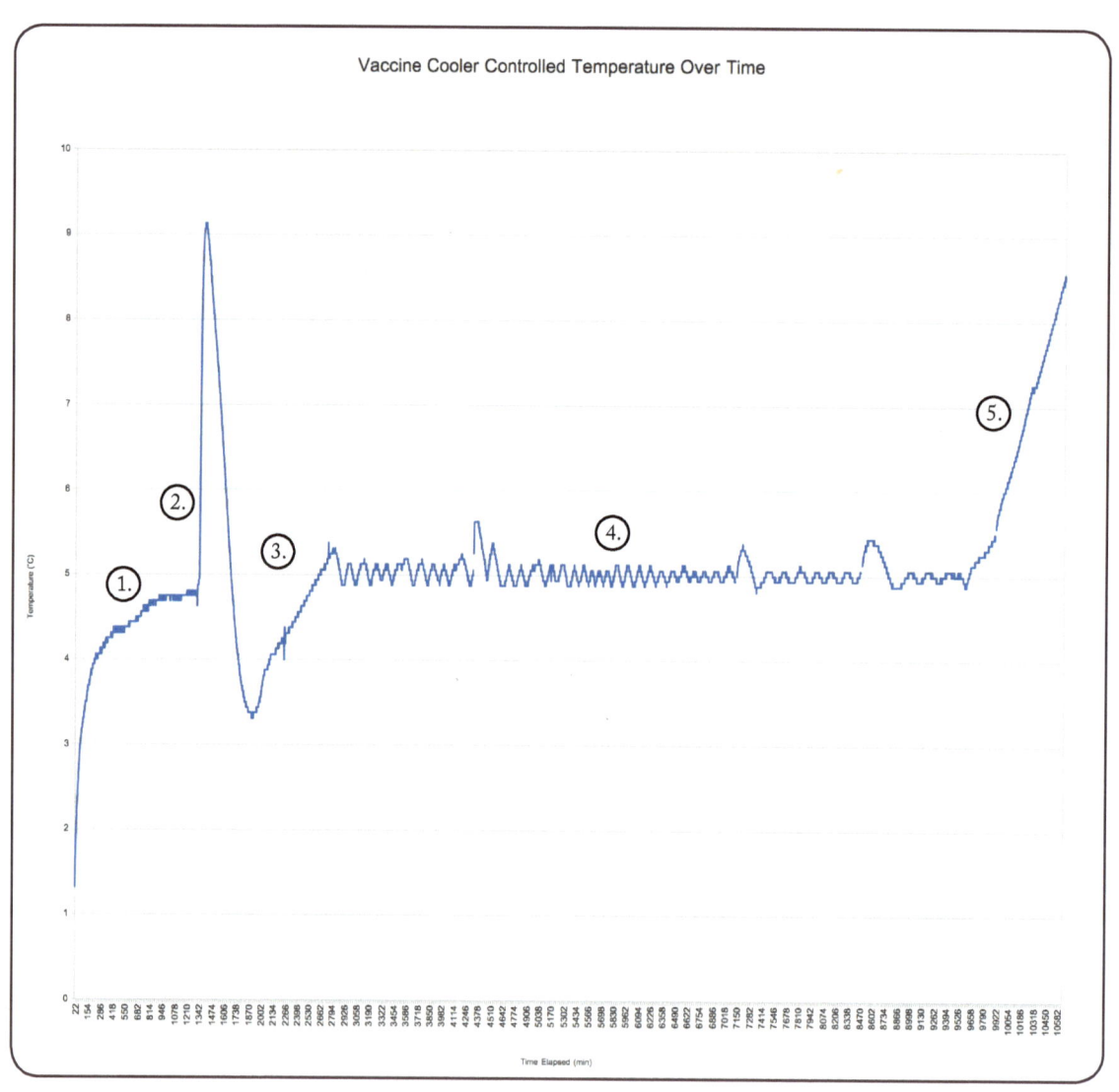

Vaccine cooler test, begun Feb. 26 2019. Phases of chart are as follows: (1.) Recovery from superchilled startup. (2.) Warm water bottles added. (3.) Thermostat reacts and settles at target temp. (4.) Hold temp. at 5°C +-0.5 for 117 hours (5.) Dry ice completely consumed, temperature rises.

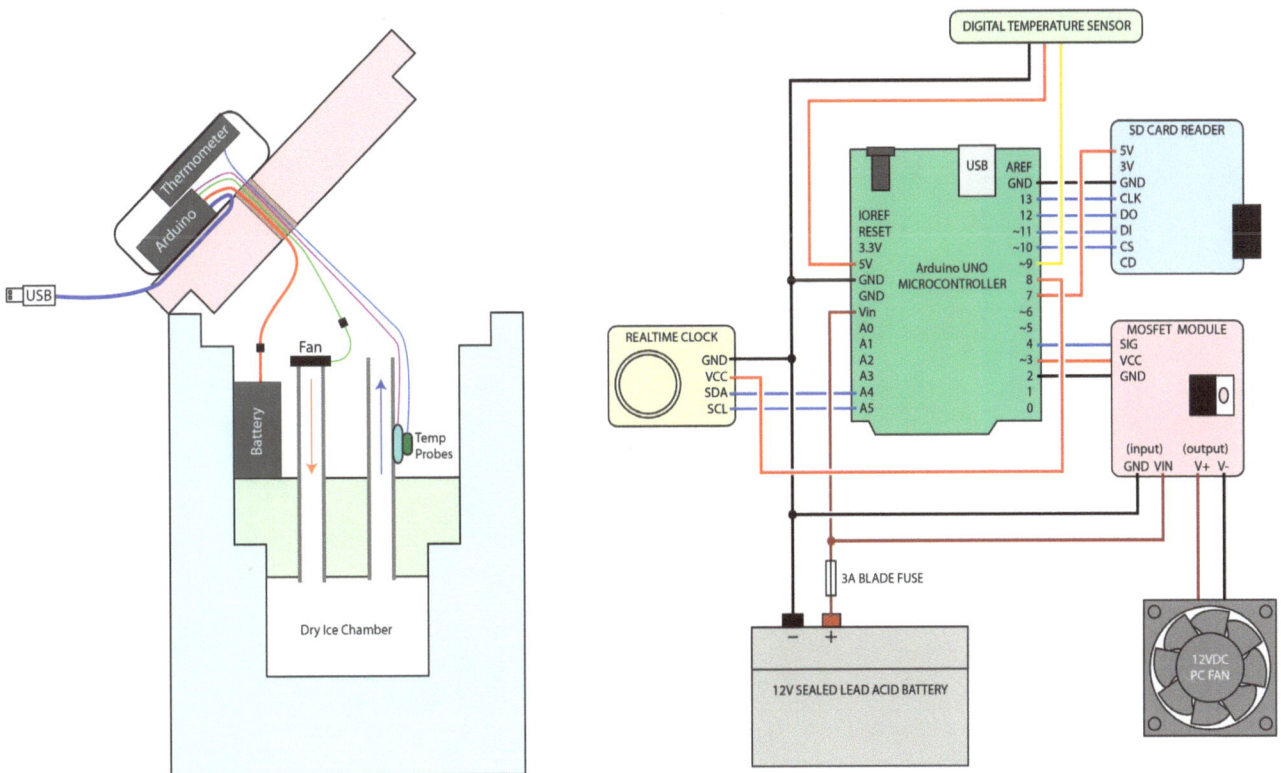

Acknowledgements

Many thanks to my wife Lindsay for her encouragement, patience, and layout skills. And for tolerating a big foam cooler in our living room for six months of R&D.

About the Author

David Hartkop is a graduate of the school of Film and Television of Loyola Marymount University, class of 2000. He has worked in commercials, feature film, and eventually found a home in the world of digital special effects. Other projects include solar coffee roasters, 3D printing with metal clay, and experiments with flying spherical cameras on drones. Hobbies include sci-fi reading, designing contraptions, running, and storytelling with dramatic flair. David lives with his wife and son in Medford, Oregon.

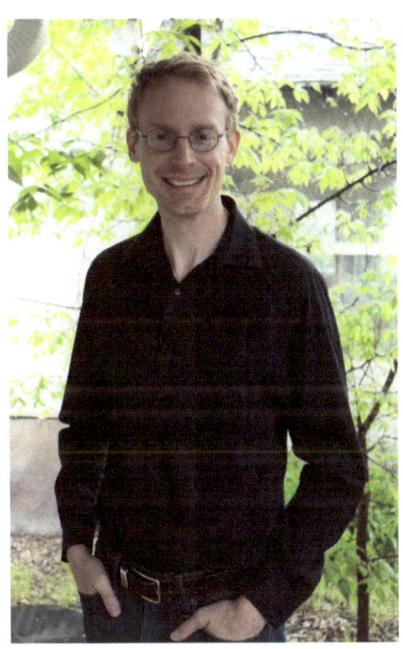